THE ROLE OF INTERLEUKIN-2 IN THE TREATMENT OF CANCER PATIENTS

The role of interleukin-2 in the treatment of cancer patients

Edited by

JOHN WAGSTAFF, MD, MB, ChB, MRCP

Senior Lecturer in Medical Oncology
Free University Hospital
Amsterdam, The Netherlands

SPRINGER SCIENCE+BUSINESS MEDIA, B.V.

Library of Congress Cataloging-in-Publication Data

The Role of interleukin-2 in the treatment of cancer patients / edited by John Wagstaff.
p. cm.
Includes bibliographical references and index.
ISBN 978-94-010-4769-2 ISBN 978-94-011-1753-1 (eBook)
DOI 10.1007/978-94-011-1753-1
1. Interleukin-2--Therapeutic use. 2. Cancer--Immunotherapy.
I. Wagstaff, John, 1952- . II. Title: Role of interleukin-two in the treatment of cancer patients.
[DNLM: 1. Interleukin-2--therapeutic uses. 2. Killer Cells--immunology. 3. Neoplasms--therapy. QZ 266 R745 1993]
RC271.I47R65 1993
616.99'406--dc20
DNLM/DLC
for Library of Congress 93-104

ISBN 978-94-010-4769-2

Printed on acid-free paper

Contents

Preface

Recombinant DNA technology has made it possible to produce human proteins on an industrial scale in highly pure form. Cytokines are proteins or glycoproteins which are responsible for mediating the hosts biological response to injury, inflammation and antigenic challenge. Many of these cytokines are intimately involved in controlling the activity of immune responses. At the beginning of the 1980's the first recombinant human cytokine, namely interferon-α_2, entered clinical trial and has subsequently been registered for use both in North America and Europe for the treatment of a number of malignant diseases. In the mid 1980's Interleukin-2 entered clinical trial and has also now been registered for the treatment of metastatic renal cell carcinoma and has promising activity in a number of other tumor types. This book has been written with the intention of providing a review of what is known of the biology and clinical activity of this interesting cytokine. The aim was to provide clinicians who are using Interleukin-2 with an overview of this cytokine and to assess its future potential. The clinical development of IL-2 has taught both the laboratory scientist and clinical researcher much about the clinical use of cytokines. These lessons are important as an increasing number of these potent molecules will be entering clinical trial in the coming years.

List of contributors

JENS ATZPODIEN
Department of Haematology & Oncology, Medical University Hannover, P.O. Box 610180, DW-3000 Hannover 61, Germany
Co-authors: Axel Schomburg and Hubert Poliwoda

JOHANNA W. BAARS
Department of Haematology, Dr Daniel den Hoed Clinic, P.O. Box 5201, 3008 AE Rotterdam, The Netherlands

REINDER L.H. BOLHUIS
Department of Medical and Tumour Immunology, Dr Daniel den Hoed Cancer Centre, P.O. Box 5201, 3008 AE Rotterdam, The Netherlands
Co-author: Gerrit Stoter

CHRISTOPHER R. FRANKS
EuroCetus B.V., P.O. Box 23023, 1100 DM Amsterdam z-o, The Netherlands
Co-author: Peter A. Palmer

LORENZ M. JOST
Department of Internal Medicine, Laboratory for Oncology, University Hospital Zürich, Häldeliweg 4, CH-8044 Zürich, Switzerland
Co-author: Rolf A. Stahel

CORNELIS J.M. MELIEF
Department of Immunohematology, University Hospital Leiden, Building 1, E3-Q, P.O. Box 9600, 2300 RC Leiden, The Netherlands
Co-author: W. Martin Kast

GIORGIO PARMIANI
Director, Division Experimental Oncology D, National Cancer Institute, Via Venezian 1, 1-20133 Milano, Italy
Co-author: Carlo Gambacorti-Passerini

SYLVIE NEGRIER
Centre Léon Bérard, 28, Rue Laënnec, F-69373 Lyon Cedex 08, France
Co-author: Thierry O. Philip

ALBERT VON ROHR
CRC Department of Medical Oncology, Christie Hospital and Holt Radium Institute, Wilmslow Road, Manchester M20 9BX, U.K.
Co-author: Nick Thatcher

JOHN WAGSTAFF
Department of Oncology, Free University Hospital, De Boelelaan 1117, PO Box 7057, 1007 MB Amsterdam, The Netherlands

1. Introduction

JOHN WAGSTAFF

> 'A disease that, starting from an insignificant injury can attack a person in prefect health, in the full vigor of early maturity, and in some insidious mysterious way, within a few months, can destroy life, is surely a subject important enough to demand our best thought and continued study.
>
> Nature often gives us hints to her profoundest secrets, and it is possible that she has given us a hint which, if we will but follow, may lead us on the solution of this difficult problem.'
>
> W.B. Coley, 1891 [1]

For over 200 years there have been reports in the cancer literature of spontaneous regressions of malignant tumours after an episode of severe infection, especially when the infectious focus was in or in the neighbourhood of the malignancy [2]. William Coley observed a complete remission of the tumour in a patient with a soft tissue sarcoma in the neck after two episodes of severe erysipelas in the same region [3]. This observation led him to explore whether he could use a filtrate of bacterial cultures, later called 'Coley's toxins', for the induction of tumour regressions. Although some dramatic 'cures' were achieved [1–4], the toxin preparations and mode of administration were variable and frequently the toxicity outweighed any antitumour efficacy and even led to a fatal outcome [4]. The clinical interest in this approach waned with the advent of radiotherapy and chemotherapy. Growing insights into the workings of the immune system and the availability of recombinant DNA technology has, however, resulted in a renewed interest immunotherapy. Several highly pure human recombinant DNA produced cytokines are now routinely used in clinical oncology and some have been shown to possess considerable efficacy. Examples include interferon alpha (IFN-a) in hairy cell leukaemia [5] and the use of haematopoeitic growth factors to enhance bone marrow recovery after chemotherapy [6]. It has become increasingly clear that these potent molecules will allow the manipulation of the immune system in

J. Wagstaff (ed.), The Role of Interleukin-2 in the Treatment of Cancer Patients, 1-5.

ways which were hitherto impossible. It may well be that cytokines are what Professor Huxley was thinking of when, in 1881, he said:

> sooner or later the pharmacologist will supply the physician with the means of affecting, in any desired sense, the function of any physiological element of the body.

In 1976, Morgan and colleagues [7] showed that normal human T lymphocytes could be cultured for extended periods, even for up to a year, in media that had been 'conditioned' by growth of phytohemagglutinin (PHA) stimulated human peripheral blood mononuclear cells. They named the factor responsible T cell growth factor (TCGF) [7]. Following the purification of TCGF, it became apparent that this agent exerted biological effects on cells other than T lymphocytes and this cytokine was, therefore, renamed interleukin-2 (IL-2) in 1979 [8].

Since then, much has been learned about this molecule. IL-2 is a glycoprotein with a molecular weight which lies between 14,500 and 17,000 Dalton with variation due to differences in glycosylation [9, 10]. Recombinant IL-2, which lacks the carbohydrate residues, is as active as natural IL-2 [10]. Glycosylation is thus not required for IL-2 activity. IL-2 consists of 133 amino-acids with a single disulphide bond between residues 58 and 105, which is essential for the activity of this cytokine [9]. IL-2 belongs to the family of cytokines, glycoproteins with a low molecular weight, which play an important role in the regulation of cell growth and differentiation, the immune response and haematopoiesis [11]. In normal circumstances, these agents are produced in minute amounts and act in a paracrine or autocrine way [11]. Thus IL-2 is not intended to be an endocrine hormone and it was, therefore, always likely that the its intravenous administration to patients would produced non-physiological effects. IL-2 is mainly produced by activated T helper cells, although activated cytotoxic T cells and an activated subset of natural killer (NK) cells are also able to secrete IL-2 under special circumstances [10].

The target cells for IL-2 are, among others, activated mature T cell populations, activated large granular lymphocytes and activated B cells [9, 10, 12]. The biological characteristics of this cytokine are such that it is unlikely to possess direct anticancer effects against solid tumours. Any antitumour effects observed in vivo must be due to induction of secondary effector systems and IL-2 can, therefore, be considered to be true biological response modifier. Characteristics, which make IL-2 attractive for use as an anticancer agent are:

1. Stimulation of proliferation of helper and cytotoxic T cells primed by antigen [9, 12, 13].
2. Induction of secretion of lymphokines such as IFN-γ and TNF [14, 15], cytokines which have been shown to have a direct antiproliferative effect [15–18].
3. Enhancement of the cytotoxicity of T- and NK cells [9, 12, 13, 19].
4. Under the influence of IL-2, a subpopulation of lymphocytes can develop 'lymphokine activated killer' (LAK) activity. LAK activity is defined

operationally as the in vitro lysis by lymphocytes of both autologous and allogeneic fresh tumour cells, as well as cultured tumour cells including these which are NK cell resistant [19–22]. The LAK cytotoxicity is non Major Histocompatibility Complex (MHC) dependent and aspecific. The majority of the lymphocytes exhibiting LAK activity are of the NK phenotype [20–22], but T lymphocytes, especially those with the gamma-delta receptor can also show LAK cytotoxicity [19]. It is better to speak of LAK activity than of the more common term LAK cells, because different subpopulations of lymphocytes can exhibit the LAK phenomenon [19].

In murine models, the intravenous injection of LAK cells induced a significant reduction in the number and size of pulmonary and hepatic metastases [23, 24]. The systemic administration of multiple high doses of IL-2 induced significant LAK cytotoxicity in vivo and was associated with the regression of fibrosarcoma and melanoma metastases, as well as irradication of disseminated murine leukaemia [25, 26]. It became clear from these studies that there existed a clear relationship between the dose of IL-2, the number of LAK cells infused and therapeutic efficacy [23–27]. Maas et al. [28] have, however, shown that low doses of IL-2 can also cure mice bearing a large burden of metastasised tumour. In their model, the enhanced cytotoxicity of lymphocytes and macrophages and the local production of cytokines such as TNF, causing tumour necrosis due to stasis of blood flow, seemed to be important for antitumour efficacy [28, 29]. Thus providing further evidence that IL-2 does not exert a direct antitumour effect, but induces it indirectly by modulating the function of the immune system [27–29].

The variety of physiological effects of IL-2 and the encouraging animal experiments led to the exploration of its usefulness as an immunotherapeutic agent for human cancer patients. IL-2, derived from the Jurkat cell line was first used for clinical studies, but this could soon be replaced by recombinant IL-2 derived from E. coli. Since the introduction of the highly pure recombinant material IL-2 has been extensively studied in the clinic and has been clearly shown to induce remissions in some human solid malignancies, especially in patients with metastatic renal cell cancer and melanoma [30–34].

The toxicities induced by systemic IL-2 treatment bear a striking resemblance to the clinical signs and symptoms observed in the early phase of septic shock or those seen after experimental endotoxin administration [30–35]. Many mediator systems, known to be involved in the pathogenesis of the clinical signs and symptoms during septic shock are also involved in the induction of IL-2 toxicity. This similarity between the two clinical entities raises the question whether IL-2 treatment, in the way that it has been frequently used, offers more benefit to the patients than endotoxin administration. In other words, apart from the standardised IL-2 preparations now available, have we more to offer than Coley did 100 years ago with his toxins? Both treatments induce a myriad reactions, including release of secondary cytokines, activation of other mediator systems such as the complement cascade and enhanced activity of the immune system. The high doses which are frequently used disturb the delicate regulation of the interplay between IL-2, its receptor and the involved immune cells which are normally activated by this cytokine. It might well be that IL-2 must be used in a more sophisticated way in order to gain the maximum benefit from the special characteristics of this cytokine. Consideration of these problems led to the idea that the time was ripe for a summary of the clinical effects of IL-2 and an appraisal of the mechanisms underlying its ability to induce remissions of tumours and induce toxicity. The aim of this book was, therefore, to provide an overview of the clinical results, insight into the biological effects of this cytokine and a discussion of its future potential. The authors have been selected from both laboratory and clinical scientists working in the field of IL-2 in Europe. The ultimate aim of the book was to attempt to provide an answer to the question posed by William Coley [36] almost 100 years ago namely:

> The question may very properly be asked, why it is that the results are so variable, that some cases yield such brilliant results while others are apparently but little benefited by the toxins? My own explanation is, that in all cases there is a certain balance of forces, the powerful proliferating tendency of the tumour cells on the one hand, and the natural resisting power of the normal cells, aided by the blood serum, on the other.

References

1. Coley WB. Contribution to the knowledge of sarcoma. Ann Surg 1891; 14: 199–221.
2. Coley Nauts H, Fowler GA, Bogatko FH. A review of the influence of bacterial infection and of bacterial products (Coley's toxins) on malignant tumors in man. Acta Med Scand 1953; (Suppl 276): 5–102 (NB 274–277 in one band!).
3. Coley WB. The treatment of malignant tumors by repeated inoculations of erysipelas: with a report of ten original cases. Am J Med Sci 1893; 105: 487–511.
4. Coley WB. Late results of the treatment of inoperable sarcoma by the mixed toxins of erysipelas and bacillus prodigiosus. Am J Med Sci 1906; 131: 375–430.
5. Balkwill FR. Interferons. In: Balkwill FR. Cytokines in Cancer Therapy. Oxford: Oxford University Press 1989: 23–53.
6. Scarffe JH. Emerging clinical uses for GM-CSF. Eur J Cancer 1991; 27: 1493–1504.
7. Morgan DA, Ruscetti FW, Gallo R. Selective in vitro growth of T lymphocytes from normal human bone marrows. Science 1976; 193: 1007–8.
8. Aarden LA, Brunner TK, Cerottini JC, et al. Revised Nomenclature for Antigen-Nonspecific T Cell Proliferation and Helper Factors. J Immunol 1979; 123; 2928–9.
9. Smith KA. Interleukin-2: Inception, Impact and Implications. Science 1988; 240: 1169–76.
10. Oppenheim JJ, Ruscetti FW, Faltynek C. Cytokines. In: Stites DP, Terr AI, editors. Basic and Clinical Immunology. Prentice Hall International Inc, 7th ed. 1991; 86–90.
11. Balkwill FR. General principles of cytokine therapy in cancer. In: Balkwill FR. Cytokines in cancer therapy. Oxford: Oxford University Press 1989; 1–7.
12. Ruscetti F.W. Interleukin-2. In: Oppenheim JJ, Shevach EM, editors. Immunophysiology. The role of Cells and Cytokines in Immunity and Inflammation. Oxford: Oxford University Press (paperback, 1st ed.) 1991; 46–66.
13. Taniguchi T, Matsui H, Fryjita T, et al. Structure and expression of a cloned cDNA for human interleukin-2. Nature 1983; 302: 305–7.
14. Mier JW, Vachino G, van de Meer JW, et al. Induction of circulating tumour necrosis factor (TNF alpha) as the mechanisms for the febrile response to Interleukin-2 (IL-2) in cancer

patients. J Clin Immunol 1988; 8: 426–36.
15. Gemlo BT, Palladino MA, Joffe HS, et al. Circulating cytokines in patients with metastatic cancer treated with recombinant Interleukin-2 and lymphokine activated killer cells. Cancer Res 1988; 48: 5864–7.
16. Ottesen SS, Ahrenkiel V, Kieler J. Recombinant human interferon-g exerts an anti-proliferative effect and modulates the expression of human leucocyte antigens A,B,C and DR in human, endothelial cell lines. Cancer Immunol Immunother 1990; 31: 93–8.
17. Le J, Vilcek J. Biology of Disease. Tumour Necrosis Factor and Interleukin-1: Cytokines with Multiple Overlapping Biological Activities. Lab Invest 1987; 56: 234–48.
18. Frei E III, Springs D. Tumour Necrosis Factor: Still a Promising Agent. J Clin Oncol 1989; 7: 291–4.
19. Bolhuis RLH, Sturm E, Braakman E. T cell targeting in cancer therapy. Cancer Immunol Immunother 1991; 34: 1–8.
20. Grimm EA, Mazumder A, Zhang HZ, Rosenberg SA. The lymphokine-activated killer cell phenomenon: lysis of NK resistant fresh solid tumour cells by IL-2 activated autologous human peripheral blood lymphocytes. J Exp Med 1982; 155: 1823–41.
21. Grimm EA, Ramsey KM, Mazumder A, et al. Lymphokine activated cell phenomenon II. The precursor phenotype is serologically distinct from peripheral T lymphocytes, memory CTL, and NK cells. J Exp Med 1983; 157: 884–97.
22. Grimm EA, Robb RJ, Roth JA, et al. Lymphokine-activated killer cell (LAK) phenomenon III. Evidence that IL-2 alone is sufficient for direct activation of PBL into LAK. J Exp Med 1983; 158: 1356–61.
23. Mulé JJ, Shu S, Schwarz SL, Rosenberg SA. Adoptive immunotherapy of established metastases with LAK cells and recombinant Interleukin 2. Science 1984; 225: 1487–9.
24. Lafreniere R, Rosenberg SA. Successful immunotherapy of murine experimental hepatic metastases with lymphokine-activated killer cells and recombinant interleukin 2. Cancer Res 1985; 45: 3735–41.
25. Rosenberg SA, Mulé JJ, Spiess PJ, et al. Regression of established pulmonary metastases and subcutaneous tumour mediated by the systemic administration of high-dose recombinant interleukin 2. J Exp Med 1985;161:1169–88.
26. Thompson JA, Peace DJ, Klarnet JP, et al. Eradication of disseminated murine leukemia with high-dose interleukin 2. J Immunol 1986; 137: 3675–80.
27. Rosenberg SA, Longo DL, Lotze MT. Principles and Applications of Biological Therapy. In: De Vita VT Jr, Hellman S, Rosenberg SA, editors. Cancer. Principles and Practice of Oncology. Philadelphia: JB Lippincott Company, 32d ed. 1989: 332–47.
28. Maas RA, Dullens HFJ, den Otter W. Mechanisms of Tumour Regressions Induced by Low Doses of Interleukin 2. In Vivo 1991; 5: 637–42.
29. De Mik HJI, Koten JW, Maas RA, et al. Tumour Regression by IL-2 Mediated Stagnation of Blood Flow. In Vivo 1991; 5: 679–84.
30. Rosenberg SA, Lotze MJ, Yang JC, et al. Experience with the use of high dose interleukin-2 in the treatment of 652 cancer patients. Ann Surg 1989; 210: 474–85.
31. West WH, Tauer KW, Yannille JR, et al. Constant-infusion recombinant interleukin-2 in adoptive immunotherapy of advanced cancer. N Eng J Med 1987; 316: 898–905.
32. Eberlein TJ, Schoof DD, Jung SE, et al. A new regimen of interleukin-2 and lymphokine activated killer cells. Efficacy without significant toxicity. Arch Int Med 1988; 148: 2571–6.
33. Wagstaff J. Lymphokines and cytokines. In: Pinedo HM, Longo DL, Chabner BA, editors. Cancer chemotherapy and biological response modifiers. Annual 12. Elsevier Science Publishers BV 1991; 165–71.
34. Rosenberg SA. Adoptive Cellular Therapy. Clinical Applications. In: De Vita VT Jr, Hellman S, Rosenberg SA. Biological Therapy of Cancer. Philadelphia: JB Lippincott Company 1991:214–36.
35. Siegel JP, Puri RK. Interleukin-2. Toxicity. J Clin Oncol 1991; 9: 694–704.
36. Coley WB. Late results of the treatment of inoperable sarcoma by the mixed toxins of erysipelas and bacillus prodigiosus. Am J Med Sci 1906; 131: 375–430.

2. Interleukin-2 as single agent

Dose, scheduling and optimum immunomodulatory dose

LORENZ M. JOST and ROLF A. STAHEL

1. Introduction

Murine models have shown dose-dependent and synergistic effects for the combination of interleukin-2 (IL-2) and ex vivo generated lymphokine-activated killer (LAK) cells in the treatment of established pulmonary metastases [1, 2]. Based on these data, a large number of clinical studies were initiated using the same technique of adoptive immunotherapy. Questions, however, arose as to whether LAK cells contributed to the therapeutic results. The initial studies done with IL-2 alone [3, 4] were therefore expanded. The results of phase I and II studies involving more than 800 patients are now available (see Tables 1–3). Unfortunately, no consensus on dose and schedule with regard to optimal immune stimulation and best tumour response has emerged.

Progress has been hindered by a lack of an understanding of the precise mechanisms of IL-2 mediated anti-tumour effect. IL-2 might mediate anti-tumour effects through diverse mechanisms including:

a) lysis by natural killer (NK)/LAK cells,
b) reversal of immune suppression by either stimulation of specific $CD4^+$ helper or primed specific $CD8^+$ cytotoxic T-lymphocytes (CTL),
c) facilitation of antibody-dependent cellular cytotoxicity (ADCC),
d) tumour cell lysis mediated by locally produced cytokines such as tumour necrosis factor or interferon-gamma, or
e) a combination of the above.

Each of these mechanisms might achieve optimal in vivo efficacy under different immunologic conditions, and the manipulation needed to achieve such efficacy might vary depending on the individual dysfunction of the immune system associated with each tumour. Furthermore, the mechanisms leading to tumour response could differ not only among patients with various cancers but probably also among patients with the same type of tumour and even among subpopulations of tumour cells within a single tumour.

The complexity of anti-tumour immune reactions is further increased by potentially opposing secondary effects of IL-2 administration. For example,

J. Wagstaff (ed.), The Role of Interleukin-2 in the Treatment of Cancer Patients, 7-28.

Table 1. Response rates in phase I and II studies of systemic IL-2 monotherapy in melanoma patients

Year	Reference	N	N with CR	N with PR	Schedule of IL-2 therapy	Cumulative dose (MIU m²) during the first 4 weeks	Cumulative dose (MIU m²) during the first 8 weeks
90	Parkinson et al. [35]	46	2	8	B.i.v. 3 × /d d1–5, 8–12	724	–
91	McCabe et al. [38]	45	2	5	B.i.v. 3 × /d d1–5, 11–15	724	–
91	Whitehead et al. [40]	42	0	4	B.i.v. 3d/w × > 6	472–720	708–1440
89	Rosenberg et al. [34]	42	0	0	B.i.v. 3 × /d 5d/w × 2	(72)–724	–
89	Allison et al. [41]	8	0	0	B.i.v. 1 × /d, 5d/w × 4	36–72	–
86	Atkins et al. [115]	3	0	0	B.i.v. 1 × /w 4 × –14 ×	0.24, 1.2, 12	0,4–72
89	Thatcher et al. [69]	31	0	4	Intrasplenically d1, B.i.v. d1,3,5,7$^{\times 1-3}$	30–660	30–990
88	Thompson et al. [48]	15	0	0	B.i.v. (2h) 3 × /d d1–5 × 4 or c.i.v. 5d/w × 4	36 or 360	–
88	Sosman et al. [47]	7	0	0	B.i.v. 1 × /d 4d/w × 4 or c.i.v. or hybrid 4d/w × 4	96 or 288	–
89	Kohler et al. [116]	3	0	0	B.i.v. 3 × /d or c.i.v. d1–7	0.007, 0.7, 70	–
90	Richards et al. [50]	33	0	3	C.i.v. d1–5, 13–17, and d21–24, 28–31	324	–
91	Perez et al. [60]	17	0	1	C.i.v. 1d/w × 8 (1–16)	72–288	144–576
88	Richards et al. [117]	12	0	0	C.i.v. 1d/w × 6	12–40	18–60
89	Creekmore et al. [61]	6	0	2	C.i.v. 1d/w × 4, 2d/w × 4	120	360
89	Goldstein et al. [118]	4	0	0	C.i.v. 4d/w × 4	48	–
88	Paciucci et al. [119]	3	0	3	C.i.v. 6d/w × 4	488	–
91	Meyers et al. [56]	13	0	0	PEG-IL-2 1 b.i.v./ w × > 4	0.8–80	1.6–160
90	Urba et al. [57]	4	0	0	i.m. 5d/w × 3	1.5–150	–
89	Mitchell et al. [37]	38	2	7	CTX + b.i.v. d1–5, 8–12 × 1–9	270–324	324–972
89	Lindemann et al. [79]	18	0	2	CTX × 3, b.i.v. 1 × /d, d1–14, 22–26, 29–33, 43–47, 50–54	180–886	180–1024
Total		390	6 (1.5%)	49 (12.6%)			

B.i.v. = bolus intravenously (10–120 min.), c.i.v. = 24h-continuous intravenous infusion, CR = complete response, CTX = cyclophosphamide, d = day, IL-2 = interleukin-2, i.m. = intramuscular, MIU/m² = 10^6 International units of IL-2 (planned dose calculated with a body weight of 70 kg and a body surface of 1.74 m²; Cetus units have been converted by a factor 6), PEG-IL-2 = Polyethylene glycol-modified IL-2, PR = partial response, Pts = patients, N = number of evaluable patients, s.c. = subcutaneous, w = week

Table 2. Response rates in phase I and II studies of systemic IL-2 monotherapy in patients with renal cell cancer

Year	Reference	N	N with CR	N with PR	Schedule of IL-2 therapy	Cumulative dose (MIU/m²) during the first 4 weeks	Cumulative dose (MIU/m²) during the first 8 weeks
89	Rosenberg et al. [34]	54	4	8	B.i.v. 3 × /d 5d/w × 2	(72–) 724	-
90	Bukowski et al. [42]	41	1	4	B.i.v. 1 × /d 3 × /w	120	240
91	McCabe et al. [38]	37	1	2	B.i.v. 3 × /d d1–5, 11–15	724	-
91	W-j. Poo et al. [120]	20	0	4	B.i.v. 3 × /d d1–5, 11–15	724	-
90	Abrams et al. [75]	16	0	0	B.i.v. d1–5, 12–16	724	-
88	Javadpour et al. [121]	10	1	2	B.i.v. d1–5 every other week	180	360
88	Sosman et al. [47]	21	0	3	B.i.v. 1 × /d 4d/w × 4 or c.i.v. or hybrid 4d/w × 4	96 or 288	-
91	Sosman et al. [59]	18	0	1	C.i.v. or hybrid 4d/w × 4, then 33–50% dose 4d/w × 4	48	64–72
88	Thompson et al. [48]	5	0	0	B.i.v. (2h) 3 × /d d1–5 × 4 or c.i.v. 5d/w × 411	36 or 360	-
89	Kohler et al. [116]	3	0	0	B.i.v. 3 × /d or c.i.v. d1–7	0.007, 0.7, 70	-
89	Negrier et al. [36]	32	2	4	C.i.v. d1–5, d12–16 × 1–6	171	171–342
89	Stoter et al. [51]	18	2	1	C.i.v. d1–5, 12–17 × 2	198	396
91	Perez et al. [60]	12	1	1	C.i.v. 1d/w × 8 (1–16)	72–288	144–576
89	Goldstein et al. [118]	9	0	0	C.i.v. 4d/w × 4	48	-
91	Ubhi et al. [28]	5	2	2	C.i.v. d1–5, 7–12	180	-
88	Paciucci et al. [119]	5	0	1	C.i.v. 6d/w × 4	488	-
88	Richards et al. [117]	4	0	0	C.i.v. 1d/w × 6	12–40	18–60
91	Meyers et al. [56]	16	0	2	PEG-IL-2 1 b.i.v./w × >4	0.8–80	1.6–160
90	Whitehead et al. [58]	15	0	0	S.c. d 1–5 every other week	45	285–405
91	Sleijfer et al. [39]	21	2	4	S.c. 5d/w × 6	306	450
89	Lindemann et al. [79]	14	0	0	CTX × 3, b.i.v.1 × /d, d1–14, 22–26, 29–33, 43–47, 50–54	180–886	180–1024
88	Kolitz et al. [74]	8	0	0	CTX × 1, 6h–infusion d5–9, 12–16, 33% dose s.c. d19–23, 26–30	80	-
Total		384	16 (4.2%)	39 (10.2%)			

For legend see Table 1

Table 3. Response rates in phase I studies of regional IL-2 therapy

Year	Reference	N	N with CR	N with PR	Tumor	Route	Daily Dose
90	Sarna et al. [92]	11	0	0	RCC/Mel/Col	Intralymphatic	0.1–23
91	Yeilding et al. [95]	6	1	0	Melanoma	Intralymphatic	0.01 or 0.1
91	Cortesina et al. [97]	20	3	3	HN	Peritumoural	0.0002–0.005
90	Squadrelli et al. [98]	14	0	3	HN	LAK & peritumoural	4.6 & 0.6–1.2
86	Lotze et al. [99]	7	0	1	Ova/Col/Mel	Intraperitoneal	1.2–252
89	Beller et al. [100]	8	0	0	Ova	Intraperitoneal	0.012–12
91	Melioli et al. [101]	6	0	0	Ova/Col/Gast	Intraperitoneal	0.6–60
89	Roth et al. [102]	29	2	2	Ova	Intraperitoneal	0.03–5
91	Eggermont et al. [104]	17	0	4	Mesothelioma	Intrapleural	0.03–36
84	Pizza et al. [107]	6	3	2	UB	Intra-/ perilesional	0.0002–0.004
89	Huland et al. [108]	5	1	n/a	UB	Intravesical perfusion	3
91	Velotti et al. [109, 110]	12	2	3	UB	Intraarterial infusion	0.03–30
Total		139	12 (8.6%)	18 (12.9%)			

[a] Cetus units were multiplied by 6 and a body weight of 70 kg or a surface area of 1.74 m^2 were assumed for calculation of the daily dose. The schedules used varied from 6 weekly injections to 56 consecutive daily doses. Listed are studies that showed at least minor tumour responses

Col = colon carcinoma, Gast = gastric carcinoma, HN = head and neck carcinoma, Mel = melanoma, Ova = ovarian carcinoma, RCC = renal cell carcinoma, UB = urinary bladder carcinoma

after in vitro short-term incubation of effector with tumour cells, NK-/LAK-mediated lysis is enhanced by the addition of IL-2 in a dose-dependent manner. In vivo, however, secondary cytokines are induced as a result of IL-2 administration. As an example, interferons may lead to an up-regulation of the major histocompatibility antigen (MHC) Class I-expression on tumour cells [5], making them more resistant to NK-mediated lysis [6]. At the same time, the increased level of MHC I (and II) expression would facilitate a specific immune-response and increase the susceptibility of tumour cells to CTL-mediated lysis [7]. Such modulations of tumour cell resistance may be irrelevant if high numbers of tumour-specific and/or non-specific suppressor cells prevent any effective anti-tumour response. Such suppressor cells have been identified in animal models as well as in patients with cancer [8–11] and may become more strongly activated during immunotherapy [12]. These cells can secrete numerous suppressive factors including prostaglandin E^2 [13], transforming growth factor-beta (TGF-beta) [14, 15], suppressin [16], $1,25(OH)^2$ vitamin D^3 [17], and most likely other mediators which have not yet been characterised [18].

2. Immunologic parameters as a guide to improvement of IL-2 based therapies

Selection of patients likely to respond to IL-2 therapy, as well as defining the optimal immunomodulatory dose and schedule of IL-2 could optimise the efficacy of IL-2 based therapies. Both tasks require the availability of simple in vitro tests or measurements that would not only reflect immune activation, but also correlate with the anti-tumour response. Great efforts have therefore been undertaken to define such tests. Table 4 lists candidate parameters known to be altered by IL-2 therapy and their potential correlation with anti-tumour effects. So far no consistent parameter has been established. The interpretation of the results has been complicated by differences in treatment schedules, the timing of measurements, and by the inclusion of patients with malignancies that have turned out to be unresponsive to IL-2. Many studies describing immunologic effects were done in series of patients with no or only limited numbers of clinically relevant tumour responses. Importantly, focussing on NK/LAK activity of peripheral blood lymphocytes, lymphocyte counts and lymphocyte subsets at baseline or, as proof of optimal immune activation during or after IL-2-based treatment, has not been helpful in the past in optimising the treatment of patients with advanced cancer. An exception is a recent study analysing patients mainly treated with IL-2 and interferon-alpha at low doses [19]. In this analysis the number of $CD56^+$ NK cells was positively correlated with the clinical outcome of therapy.

The lytic capacity of retransfused, in vitro activated tumour infiltrating lymphocytes (TIL) against autologous tumour, but not against the NK- and LAK-cell sensitive K562 and Daudi cell lines, has been reported to correlate with anti-tumour response in melanoma patients [20] and implies a role for MHC-restricted cytotoxic T-lymphocytes.

Posttreatment expression of MHC Class II antigens on the tumour cells [21] might be a helpful prognostic marker. This would, however, be impossible to measure in all cases and would reveal information only after a first cycle of IL-2 treatment. Changes in expression of MHC antigens may help to trigger autoimmune reactions such as vitiligo, hypoadrenalism, autoimmune haemolytic anaemia or thyroid dysfunction possibly due to autoimmune thyroiditis [22–25]. Such parameters may reveal prognostic information, but only considerable time after the initiation of the immunotherapy. More recent studies regarding thyroid dysfunction, which is especially common after prolonged combined treatment with IL-2 and interferon-alpha, have not demonstrated a correlation with response [26, 27]. The observation of autoimmune phenomena and changes in MHC antigen expression indicate that CTL-mediated lysis may constitute the central mechanism of IL-2 induced anti-

Table 4. Response-predictive power of immunologic parameters for IL-2 based therapies

a) Pretreatment

Parameter	Tumour effect	Correlation with tumour response
Lymphocyte count	↓	Few pos. studies [122], mostly none [36, 69, 123, 124]
Number and percentage of NK cells	↓	Not systematically tested
NK/LAK activity	↓	None established [118]
Anti-CD3 stimulated Lysis	↓	Possible [28]

b) During and/or after first treatment cycle

Parameter	IL-2 effect	Correlation with tumour response
Rebound lymphocytosis	↑	Few pos. studies [122], mostly none [36, 69, 123, 124]
Eosinophilia (PBL)	↑	None established [69], trend found in [125]
Local eosinophil counts	↑	Speculative [108]
IL-2R (p55 on $CD3^+$ PBL)	↑	None established [63]
CD4/CD8 ratio	↓	None established [63, 125]
Number and percentage of NK cells	↑	Mostly none [59, 125], one positive study [19]
NK activity	↑	None established [37, 59, 125, 126]
LAK activity	↑	Not systematically tested
Mitogen-induced proliferation	↑	One positive study [127]
- Tumour Necrosis Factor	↑	One positive [127], one negative [49] study
- Interferon-gamma	↑	None established [49]
- IL-6	↑	Not systematically tested
- Soluble IL-2R	↑	None established [19, 79]
- ACTH/Cortisol	↑	Not tested, theoretically negative [65, 128]
- TGF-beta	↑	Not tested, theoretically negative
Lymphatic tumour infiltration	↑	Possibly positive [30, 129]
MHC II expression in tumours	↑	Possibly positive [21, 45]
Thyroiditis/Hypothyroidism	↑	Positive [22–25], negative [26, 27]

ACTH = adrenocorticotropic hormone, ADCC/LDCC = antibody/lectin dependent cellular cytotoxicity, IL-2R = interleukin-2 receptor, MHC = major histocompatibility complex, NK = natural killer cell, PBL = peripheral blood lymphocytes, TGF = transforming growth factor

tumour response. In accordance with this hypothesis, the only pretreatment test claimed to be predictive for responses has been the measurement of the lytic capacity of peripheral blood lymphocytes which can be induced by anti-CD3 stimulation in vitro [28]. But the small number of patients involved and the fact that the only patients achieving a complete remission belonged to the favourable prognostic group, clearly demands further confirmation.

The prognostic potential of serum levels of interleukin-1, tumour necrosis factor (TNF), and other secondary cytokines is not yet clear. If the increase in TNF serum levels should turn out to be a solid predictive marker, this would suggest an in vivo role for TNF in mediating tumour response of IL-2-based therapies despite the inefficacy of TNF as a monotherapy [29, 30]. Speculations that the IL-2-associated toxicity could be mitigated by inhibiting secreted TNF with neutralising antibodies or by specific blockade of the TNF secretion, e.g., with pentoxifylline [31, 32], thalidomide or its non-teratogenic analogues that are being developed [33], are hazardous until it is determined whether they compromise the efficacy of IL-2 based therapies.

Remarkably, reliable data are entirely lacking for the more easily obtainable parameters, such as C-reactive protein or beta$_2$-microglobulin, which are thought to reflect the overall degree of immune stimulation. Baseline suppressor activity could be another parameter which warrants further evaluation.

3. Tumour response as guide for optimising systemic IL-2 treatment

Since reliable immune parameters for monitoring and optimising treatment with biological response modifiers are not available, we can only rely on anti-tumour responses. Tables 1 and 2 list the studies which used systemic IL-2 as a single agent in the treatment of advanced, metastatic melanoma and renal cell carcinoma, the tumour types most responsive to IL-2. Since phase I studies are included, the overall activity of IL-2 as a single agent is very low and may not reflect its true potential. The listed results seem to favour the usage of short cycles with high-dose bolus-injections of IL-2. This conclusion will be discussed in the following paragraphs.

3.1. The dose dependence of tumour responses

Overall response rates for metastatic malignant melanoma and renal cell carcinoma consistently range between 18 and 24% when only phase II studies with more than 30 patients [34–37] are considered. These results have been confirmed in a phase III multi-centre study comparing IL-2 with IL-2/LAK [38]. All of these studies used a schedule similar to that employed in Rosenberg's initial IL-2/LAK studies with two cycles of high-dose IL-2 administered intravenously within 3 weeks. Complete remissions (CR) have been described almost exclusively with this approach using IL-2 doses at or near the maximal tolerated dose. The exception is a preliminary report in which subcutaneous injections of IL-2 were given for 6 weeks at moderate doses [39]. In phase I studies utilising less frequent and/or lower doses of IL-2 much lower rates of partial responses (PR) were observed along with more moderate side effects [40–42]. Based on data from patients with advanced tumours, high systemic IL-2 doses near the maximal tolerated dose are more likely to result in regressions of advanced tumours but at a considerable cost in terms of toxicity.

3.2. The effect of schedule and route on tumour responses

Disadvantages of intravenous bolus injection of high IL-2 doses, such as severe hypotension mandating close monitoring and the relatively frequent catheter-associated bacterial infections [43, 44] led to the exploration of alternative schedules and routes. Continuous intravenous infusion of IL-2 is not associated with fluctuating hypotension and makes the IL-2 treatment feasible even in an outpatient setting. The maximal tolerated dose seems, however, to be reduced to approximately one third of the daily dose given as bolus injections [45, 46]. The immune stimulation achieved by continuous intravenous infusions as measured by rebound lymphocytosis, lymphocyte subset analysis, and NK/LAK activity are equivalent or clearly superior to bolus injections of IL-2 [45, 47, 48], but secretion of secondary cytokines may be lower than with bolus injections [49]. The response rates at nearly equitoxic doses and with comparable schedules seem to be lower for continuous intravenous infusion of IL-2 than for bolus administration [50, 51], with an exception being the multicentre study reported by Negrier [36]. This has also been documented in IL-2/LAK studies with melanoma patients [52]. A possible explanation for such differences between tolerance and efficacy is that continuously high IL-2 plasma levels may suppress crucial immune reactions, such as the secretion of short-lived secondary cytokines and the trafficking of activated cells into the tumour, which might be more successfully triggered by only short IL-2 plasma peaks. Selective migration of effector cells into tumour deposits may depend exclusively on local alterations of the endothelium within the tumour as well as transendothelial gradients of cytokines and chemotactic factors [53], all of which could be disturbed if constantly high plasma levels of IL-2 lead to long-lasting generalised stimulation of endothelial cells. Such an inhibition by high intravascular cytokine levels has recently been demonstrated for intravascular interleukin-8 in respect to transendothelial migration of granulocytes [54, 55].

Prolongation of the very short half-life of intravenously injected IL-2 has been attempted by its conjugation to polyethylene glycol. Polyethylene glycol-conjugated IL-2 has shown some clinical anti-tumour activity in a phase I protocol in renal cell cancer patients [56] and will ultimately require comparison against 24-h infusions of conventional IL-2 with programmable pumps which allow varying delivery rates.

Intramuscular IL-2 injections have shown immune modulatory effects but no responses in one small phase I study [57]. Subcutaneous injections would reduce the risk of catheter-associated bacterial infections and are most suitable for use in outpatients, but high doses at present require rather impractical large volumes. A phase I study with escalation to moderate doses resulted in no tumour responses [58], while another study using higher doses showed promising responses but also considerable systemic toxicity [39]. The observed high incidence of anti-IL-2 antibody formation [58] may lead to increased neutralisation of the biological activity of the injected IL-2 over time.

In conclusion, and based on experiences derived from various phase I and II studies, it appears that systemic IL-2 should be primarily given intravenously until the favourable results for subcutaneous injections found by Sleijfer et al. [39] can be confirmed by others.

3.3. The effect of the duration of IL-2 therapy on tumour responses

A number of studies have tried to avoid the problems associated with high IL-2 doses given within short periods of time by extending the duration of the treatment while using lower doses [48, 58–60]. Repetition of treatment cycles with IL-2 alone, or with combinations of IL-2 and LAK cells or interferon-alpha, resulted in an increase of immune parameters including lymphocytosis and absolute numbers of circulating NK cells [61]. Other parameters such as NK or LAK activity and serum levels of TNF-alpha showed decremental gains with each cycle and even a decline to below pre-treatment levels [62–64]. This down-regulation may be explained by a stronger increase in the levels of corticotropin releasing hormone (CRH), adrenocorticotropic hormone (ACTH), and cortisol. After repeat cycles of IL-2 cortisol levels may reach more than 20-fold the levels found in patients with Cushing's syndrome! [65].

Elevated levels of neuroendocrine hormones following IL-2 therapy may have effects other than just down-regulation of the immune system. An autocrine or paracrine inflammatory action of ACTH [66] and CRH [67] at *low local* concentrations has recently been recognised. ACTH has mixed effects including inhibition of interferon-production and increase of tumour necrosis factor-secretion from freshly isolated or interferon-stimulated monocytes/macrophages. Low concentrations of CRH increase IL-2 receptor expression, induce leukocytes to secrete interleukin-1, β-endorphin, ACTH and alpha-melanocyte stimulating hormone and enhance lymphocyte proliferation. However, at *high concentrations* in plasma and in the central nervous system CRH acts as a coordinator of the stress response and stimulates the potent suppressive CRH-ACTH-cortisol axis. Immune stimulation at all but massive levels of IL-2 may be abrogated by the influence of this suppression.

The hypothesis that moderate doses of IL-2 are insufficient to maintain the immune activation reached after an induction cycle has been confirmed in a recent study [59]. A first group of patients was treated with a maintenance therapy of continuous infusions of IL-2 at a quarter of the induction dose. During this treatment the patients were unable to preserve the previously reached lytic activity against NK and LAK target cells. A second group of patients was treated with a reinduction cycle after 2 months of maintenance therapy with IL-2 at one third of the induction dose given as bolus injections. Again, before the reinduction cycle lytic activity was lower than after the induction cycle but did, however, increase after reinduction. Despite increased lytic activity no improvement in response rates has been observed in the second group. Future studies of combinations of IL-2 with other biological response modifiers will have to carefully address not only the question of down-regulation with repeated or extended treatment cycles but also whether the specific combination treatment leads to earlier or stronger down-regulation in vivo [68] thereby abrogating potential initial synergistic effects.

So far, the clinical results do not seem to support the need for extended or repeated treatments. In all of the studies listed in Tables 1–3, most of the responses were seen within 1 to 2 months after initiating IL-2-based therapies. In some of the early responding patients it took more than 2 months to establish maximal anti-tumour effect. In some of the early responding patients it took more than two months to establish the maximal anti-tumour effect. In such cases the best response may have been reached considerably after cessation of IL-2 based therapy [37, 69]. Later responses (after up to 4 months) have occurred rarely and only with schedules using a low frequency of IL-2 administration [42]. Prolonged treatment with regimens using high initial dose-intensity in non-responding patients with advanced cancer is therefore not warranted.

The interval between IL-2-based treatment courses may have to be extended beyond the currently used length in order to ensure optimal restimulation. Not only disappearance of side effects may be required, but restoration of unperturbed immune and neuroendocrine systems, potentially at a more favourable steady state than before treatment. This strategy would circumvent activating negative feedback loops, which otherwise might abrogate the beneficial effects of retreatment with IL-2 [63, 64]. Complete abatement of negative feedbacks such as the CRH-ACTH-Cortisol axis and the synthesis of prostaglandin E_2 by monocytes [13, 70–72] as well as the production of transforming growth factor-beta by tumour cells, monocytes, and activated T-cells (reviewed in [73]) probably needs more than 3–4 weeks even though in vitro measured NK/LAK activity returns to near baseline within days.

3.4. The modulation of the secondary effects of IL-2 responses

Efforts have been made to prevent the relatively rapid decline in immune activation following IL-2 administration. Concomitant treatment with prostaglandin synthesis inhibitors (mainly indomethacin) increases the degree and duration of immune stimulation probably by delaying the monocyte-mediated negative feedback loops described above. Indomethacin has been incorporated into most protocols in order to control side effects [42, 47, 74, 75]. Clinical and immunological data characterising the contribution of prostaglandin synthesis inhibitors are therefore currently lacking.

Theoretically, antagonists of type-II histamine receptors (e.g., cimetidine) may be beneficial for their reported ability to inhibit generation of suppressor T-cells [76–78]. H_2-receptor effects are, however, transient, and cimetidine has only been used in a uncontrolled manner to prevent stress ulcers [42, 75].

Several studies have investigated the effect of pretreatment with non-cytotoxic doses of cyclophosphamide to selectively reduce the number of suppressor T-cells before starting IL-2 or IL-2/LAK treatment. Besides one optimistic report [37], cyclophosphamide pretreatment failed to consistently demonstrate improved tumour responses in 2 smaller studies with IL-2 as a single agent [74, 79].

The hypothesis that schedules utilising high-dose bolus-injections of systemic IL-2 are optimal still needs further proof. Especially, the premises which are valid for patients with advanced tumours may differ from those applicable to patients without advanced disease who are less likely to have high levels of tumour-specific and non-specific immune suppression that may interfere with the treatment. Usage of IL-2 in an adjuvant setting as well as in combination with other potent biological response modifiers or cytostatic drugs will have to be systematically tested and should include various dose levels, schedules and routes – a task not yet accomplished.

3.5. IL-2 after autologous bone marrow transplantation (ABMT)

A promising application of IL-2 is emerging in the setting of high-dose chemo- or chemoradiotherapy followed by bone marrow transplantation. It has long been recognised that despite timely recovery of myelopoiesis and the total number of circulating lymphocytes, immunodeficiency persists for at least one year after autologous marrow transplantation [80]. The persistent immune dysfunctions observed in marrow transplant patients may impair the elimination of minimal residual disease after bone marrow transplantation and thereby contribute to the high relapse rate seen despite the increased doses of cytostatic drugs that can be delivered with this type of therapy. The immune dysfunction is marked by imbalances of helper and suppressor T-cells [81, 82], deficits in stimulated secretion of IL-2 and interferon-gamma [83, 84], deficient proliferative responses to mitogens, and diminished capacity of T-cell colony formation. In vitro, addition of IL-2 restores these defects [85]. In this state of 'cytokine deficiency', IL-2 with its broad immunostimulatory activities would appear to be a ideal therapeutic modality. Although some in vitro studies have described myelo-suppressive effects of IL-2 [86], it has been shown in phase I studies that infusions of IL-2 at cumulative doses ranging from 1.5–22.5 MIU/m^2 over 3–5 days can be safely given after autologous bone marrow transplantation. Such consolidative IL-2 therapy enhances the marrow regeneration by inducing messenger RNA for and secretion of multiple haematopoietic growth factors [87], restores the deficient production of IL-2 and interferon-gamma [83], and accelerates the recovery of the number and activity of NK cells [88, 89]. Even in post-transplant patients without IL-2 treatment an early rise in the percentage of NK cells among peripheral lymphocytes can be seen. This increase may, however, not translate into significant cytolytic activity against residual tumour cells because of low levels of supportive cytokines produced by other mononuclear cells.

Exogenous substitution of IL-2 at low doses may reconstitute the immune defects associated with bone marrow transplantation. This should reduce the increased rate of post-transplant viral infections and induce significant non-MHC restricted anti-tumour cytotoxicity at that crucial time of minimal residual disease, thereby hopefully reducing the relapse rate. In this setting, even prolonged treatment with IL-2 may be possible without eliciting strong down-regulation, partially because of the low number of monocytes seen early after bone marrow transplantation.

Preliminary results with daily infusions of IL-2 at 0.2 MIU/m²/day over 3 months were found to be immunologically effective and safe even in patients after rescue with allogeneic T-cell depleted bone marrow [90]. A 15-fold increase in numbers of circulating NK cells was seen after 9 weeks of therapy with little change in the absolute number of circulating T-lymphocytes and a notable absence of any signs of enhanced graft-versus-host disease. Large controlled studies will, however, be necessary to establish the minimal effective dose as well as duration and schedule of administration able to prevent the frequent relapses of haematological malignancies after bone marrow transplantation. Prime attention has to be directed at avoiding the troublesome side effects of IL-2 such as fatigue, weight loss, and especially increased susceptibility to bacterial infections [43, 44] and the possibility of enhanced graft-versus-host disease after allogeneic bone marrow transplantation.

4. The regional application of IL-2

The modest response rates and the associated severe toxicities seen with conventional high-dose IL-2 regimens have triggered multiple phase I studies (summarised in Table 3) utilising regional IL-2 delivery. These studies have been aimed at restricting the distribution of IL-2 (and LAK cells) to the tumour site in order to achieve high local concentrations with less systemic side effects.

As will be discussed in the following paragraphs, regional IL-2 may lead to remarkable clinical responses, especially when applied into defined cavities, where lasting local IL-2 levels can be maintained with low cumulative doses of injected IL-2 and without leading to elevated systemic cytokine levels. High intracavitary doses of IL-2 may lead to unnecessary local and systemic toxicity similar to that seen with continuous intravenous infusion of IL-2 because of constant resorption of IL-2 and may promote local down-regulation of immune effector cells due to excessively high local IL-2 levels. Regional IL-2 injections are therefore unlikely to require maximum tolerable doses of IL-2 for optimal tumour responses.

4.1. Intralymphatic IL-2

Infusions into the lymphatic vessels of the foot were used in patients with renal cell carcinoma based on the hypothesis that this may lead to enhanced immunologic activity in the hilar lymph nodes. At low cumulative doses (approx. 1–5 MIU/m²), a greater activation of killer cells from renal hilar lymph nodes could be seen compared to peripheral blood lymphocytes [91]. At higher doses, pharmacokinetics, immunomodulatory, and side effects resemble those of intravenous application of IL-2 because of rapid entry of the IL-2 into the circulation. In patients with various other tumours, intralymphatic injections of IL-2 doses > 1 MIU/m²/day have shown immunomodulatory effects but no major clinical responses [92, 93]. As seen with IL-2 delivered subcutaneously [94], a greater number of patients develop antibodies against IL-2 (42%) compared to intravenous IL-2 (16%) [92]. Preliminary results of a study using first a 5-day cycle of infusions into lymph nodes with metastatic tumour deposits followed by 2 cycles of regional intradermal injections in patients with local and regional metastatic melanoma showed 1 CR among 6 patients treated at the lowest 2 dose levels (0.01 and 0.1 MIU/day) [95].

4.2. Peritumoural IL-2

Locally metastatic head and neck tumours have been treated with regional injections of natural IL-2 derived from Jurkat cells (200–5000 U/day for 10 days) [96, 97]. Among 20 patients, 3 CR, 3 PR, and 7 minor responses lasting 2–10 months have been reported despite only minor changes in systemic immune parameters. This schedule was non-toxic and, if confirmed, would be at least as effective as a schedule using up to 100-fold higher IL-2 doses in conjunction with regionally administered LAK cells (3 PR and 3 minor responses among 14 patients) [98]. Further documentation of the activity of IL-2 given by this route is awaited from several trials.

4.3. Intraperitoneal IL-2

The intraperitoneal application of IL-2 in patients with ovarian carcinoma, tumours of the gastrointestinal tract or melanoma has been studied by several groups [99–101]. Pharmacokinetic data showed, that low doses of IL-2 result in high intraperitoneal IL-2 levels with concomitantly low serum concentrations. Severe local toxicity such as painful sterile or bacterial peritonitis with enhanced ascites production, peritoneal fibrosis and enhanced adhesions made this route cumbersome when higher IL-2-doses of up to 70 MIU/m²/day were applied during 5 to 7 days. Furthermore, systemic toxicity [99] similar to that seen with intravenous IL-2 developed at these higher dose levels. For a schedule using 14 days of IL-2 applications, a maximal tolerable dose of 1.0 MIU/m²/day has been defined [101]. The longer persistence of IL-2 in the ascites compared to serum levels, cell counts and results of cytokine and cytotoxicity measurements favour injection of only the minimally effective dose (0.03–0.1 MIU/m²/day) for further studies. In a recently closed phase I–II study in patients with ovarian carcinoma, 2 CR out of 10 patients treated at the lowest dose level (0.12 MIU/m²/day during 16 or 56 dys) have been surgically documented [102]. Both responding patients had minimal residual disease prior to treatment and all patients at this dose level had negligible IL-2 serum levels and side effects. The inclusion of additional patients at increased IL-2 dose levels has not documented a dose-dependent pattern of tumour response. Only 2 further partial remissions among a total of 19 patients were seen. The study confirmed the considerable local toxicity of IL-2 at higher doses (> 1 MIU/day) with peritonitis and catheter-related problems which precluded completion of the planned schedule in most patients (B. Lembersky, personal communication).

4.4. Intrahepatic IL-2

Administration of IL-2 via the portal vein or the hepatic artery in patients with liver metastases or hepatocellular carcinoma has been described only in combination with LAK cells. Given the high volume of blood perfusing the liver, IL-2 is not likely to achieve sustained high local concentrations when used as a single agent at doses without systemic side effects.

4.5. Intrapleural IL-2

In phase I protocols, intrapleural IL-2 injections have been administered mainly to patients with mesothelioma either combined with continuous intravenous IL-2 infusion [103] or intrapleurally alone [104]. In this latter study, considerable systemic side effects including major infectious complications occurred at the highest dose level (36 MIU/day given from day 1 to 14 every month). All responses (4/17 PR, lasting 5–20 months) and 4 of 5 patients with stable disease were seen at the lowest 3 dose levels (0.003–3 MIU/day) with negligible systemic side effects. The lack of a dose-response as well as persistently high levels of IL-2 and tumour necrosis factor in the pleural fluid (without concomitantly detectable serum levels) at low injected doses of IL-2 showed that the minimal effective and the optimal intrapleural IL-2 dose are well below the maximal tolerated dose.

4.6. Regional IL-2 for bladder cancer

Bladder cancer is one of the few tumours which has shown positive results with the application of BCG (Bacille Calmette-Guérin) [105, 106] and was therefore a reasonable candidate for early studies using regional IL-2. Patients with locally advanced tumours have been treated with intralesional IL-2 injections [107], intravesical IL-2 perfusions [108], and intra-arterial IL-2 infusions [109] at various dose levels. Repeated intralesional applications of an IL-2 preparation from a xenogeneic lymphoblastoid cell line required an injection dose of more than 2000 U to result in tumour regressions [107] (N = 6, 3 CR, 2 PR), suggesting the existence of a critical local IL-2 concentration necessary to overcome the local immune inhibition. A role for the xenogeneic protein per se in mediating the observed response could be ruled out by including a control group receiving the same amount of protein with only very low IL-2 activity.

Technically even less demanding are intravesical perfusions with IL-2 which can be done after partial transurethral resection (TUR). The study of Huland and Huland [108] using natural human IL-2 (2 cycles of 3 MIU/day from day 1 to 5) documented 1 long-lasting CR among 5 patients after incomplete TUR which made determination of partial responses a problem. A high percentage of eosinophils among the urinary leukocytes was observed that did not correlate well with the degree of the eosinophilia found in the peripheral blood but might be associated with the tumour response since the patient having a CR had the highest urine eosinophil counts. Cytospins obtained from urine of different patients showed degranulated eosinophils in close contact to the tumour cells suggesting a possible role in the antitumoural mechanism. Side effects were negligible as seen with intralesional application.

Continuous intra-arterial infusions of recombinant IL-2 (0.018–18 MIU/m^2 given from day 1 to 5 and 8 to 12) into the internal iliac artery were effective (N = 12, 2 CR, 3 PR) [109, 110] but are technically more demanding and associated with dose-dependent moderate systemic side effects as seen with intravenous IL-2 infusions. Dose-dependent changes in a variety of local, immunohistological and systemic immune parameters have been observed, but did not correlate with tumour regression. The degree of eosinophilic infiltration within the tumour was low compared to the findings in cytospins obtained from patients with intravesical natural IL-2. Changes in numbers of NK cells in the blood and in situ were not seen except at the highest dose level, whereas the responses occurred at 0.18 and 1.8 MIU/m^2/day.

4.7. Intrathecal IL-2 in patients with leptomeningeal cancer

Twelve patients were treated with rather high doses (2 cycles of 6–12 MIU/day during 2 days/week) of intraventricular IL-2 administered through an Ommaya reservoir [111]. Only 1 patient tolerated this schedule. Side effects, including symptoms of increased cranial pressure associated with a strong polymorphonuclear and later lymphatic infiltration, required reductions in dose and/or frequency. Two patients showed neurologic improvement and 9 had clearance of tumour cells from spinal fluid samples. Low doses might have been more effective in these patients.

In summary, preliminary data of regional IL-2 usage show remarkable clinical responses but the optimal schedules have yet to be defined. Further studies of the mechanism responsible for tumour regressions are needed and future protocols should ask for inclusion of more patients into the dose level first associated with mild toxicity, the previous 2 dose levels and, maybe, into additional dose levels interposed in between in order to define the minimal and the optimally effective doses of regional IL-2.

5. Future prospects for IL-2 as a single agent

It has been questioned whether IL-2 as a single agent has any advantages over alternative immunologic or cytostatic therapies when applied at reasonably well tolerated doses as an outpatient therapy. Even for patients with advanced malignant renal cell carcinoma and malignant melanoma, IL-2 alone may not be significantly more efficient than high-dose interferon therapy [112, 113] or newer multi-drug combination therapies [114] respectively. Currently, randomised trials comparing these treatments are not available. If performed in the future, they should not only address the question of tumour shrinkage but also overall survival and quality of life during and after the treatment. It may well be that IL-2 as a single agent finds its best place in some well defined local therapies and in systemic use at lower doses in an adjuvant setting, such as after autologous bone marrow transplantation and complete resection of melanoma and renal cell cancer, or for enhancing immune competence after conventional chemotherapy. The potential of IL-2 in combination with other modalities will be discussed in the following chapters.

References

1. Mulé JJ, Shu S, Schwarz SL, Rosenberg SA. Adoptive immunotherapy of established pulmonary metastases with LAK cells and recombinant interleukin-2. Science 1984; 225: 1487–9.
2. Rosenberg SA, Mulé JJ, Spiess PJ, et al. Regression of established pulmonary metastases and subcutaneous tumor mediated by the systemic administration of high-dose recombinant interleukin 2. J Exp Med 1985; 161: 1169–88.
3. Lotze MT, Chang AE, Seipp CA, et al. High dose recombinant interleukin-2 in the treatment of patients with disseminated cancer: Responses, treatment-related morbidity, and histologic findings. J Am Med Assoc 1986; 256: 3117–24.
4. Rosenberg SA, Lotze MT, Muul LM, et al. A progress report on the treatment of 157 patients with advanced cancer using lymphokine-activated killer cells and interleukin-2 or high-dose interleukin-2 alone. N Engl J Med 1987; 316(15): 889–97.
5. Carrel S, Schmidt-Kessen A, Giuffrè L. Recombinant interferon-gamma can induce the expression of HLA-DR and -DQ on DR-negative melanoma cells and enhance the expression of HLA-ABC and tumor-associated antigens. Eur J Immunol 1985; 15: 118–23.
6. Trinchieri G, Perussia B. Biology of Disease. Human natural killer cells: biologic and pathologic agents. Lab Invest 1984; 50: 489–513.
7. Vanky F, Wang P, Patarroyo M, Klein E. Expression of the adhesion molecule ICAM-1 and major histocompatibility complex class I antigens on human tumor cells is required for their interaction with autologous lymphocytes in vitro. Cancer Immunol Immunother 1990; 31: 19–27.
8. Chakraborty NG, Twardzik DR, Sivanandham M, et al. Autologous melanoma-induced activation of regulatory T cells that suppress cytotoxic response. J Immunol 1990; 145(7): 2359–64.
9. Ting CC, Rodrigues D. Tumor cell-triggered macrophage-mediated suppression of the T-cell cytotoxic response to tumor associated antigens. I. Characterization of the cell components for induction of suppression. J Natl Cancer Inst 1982; 69(4): 867–72.
10. Ting CC, Hargove ME. Tumor cell-triggered macrophage-mediated suppression of the T-cell cytotoxic response to tumor associated antigens. II. Mechanisms for induction of suppression. J Natl Cancer Inst 1982; 69(4): 873–8.
11. Nakano E, Iwasaki A, Seguchi T, et al. Concanavalin A-induced suppressor cell activity in patients with renal cell carcinoma. Cancer 1991; 68: 2586–90.
12. Ebihara T, Koyama S, Fukao K, et al. Lymphokine-activated suppressor (LAS) cells in patients with gastric carcinoma. Cancer Immunol Immunother 1989; 28(3): 218–24.
13. Webb DR, Nowowiejski I. Control of suppressor cell activation via endogenous prostaglandin synthesis: the role of T cells and macrophages. Cell Immunol 1981; 63: 321–8.
14. Brown TJ, Lioubin MN, Marquardt H. Purification and characterization of cytostatic

lymphokines produced by activated human T lymphocytes. Synergistic antiproliferative activity of transforming growth factor Beta-1, interferon-gamma, and oncostatin M for human melanoma cells. J Immunol 1987; 139(9): 2977–83.
15. Rueda F, Pinol G, Gonzalez-Garrigues M, et al. Transforming growth factor release by human tumor cell lines and their interactions with other growth factors. Anticancer Res 1989; 9: 1245–8.
16. LeBoeuf RD, Carr DJJ, Green MM, Blalock JE. Cellular effects of suppressin: A biological response modifier cell of the immune system. Progr NeuroEndocrin Immunol 1990; 3(3): 176–87.
17. Koren R, Liberman UA, Maron L, et al. 1,25-Dihydroxyvitamin D_3 acts directly on human lymphocytes and interferes with the cellular response to interleukin-2. Immunopharmacology 1989; 18: 187–94.
18. Bugis SP, Lotzová E, Savage HE, et al. Inhibition of lymphokine-activated killer cells generation by blocking factors in sera of patients with head and neck cancer. Cancer Immunol Immunother 1990; 31: 176–81.
19. Haenninen EL, Koerfer A, Hadam M, et al. Biological monitoring of low-dose interleukin-2 in humans: Soluble interleukin-2 receptors, cytokines, and cell surface phenotypes. Cancer Res 1991; 50: 6312–6.
20. Aebersold P, Hyatt C, Johnson S, et al. Lysis of autologous melanoma cells by tumor-infiltrating lymphocytes: Association with clinical response. J Natl Cancer Inst 1991; 83(13): 932–7.
21. Rubin JT, Elwood LJ, Rosenberg SA, Lotze MT. Immunohistochemical correlates of response to recombinant interleukin-2-based immunotherapy in humans. Cancer Res 1989; 49: 7086–92.
22. Atkins M, Mier JW, Parkinson DR, et al. Hypothyroidism after treatment with interleukin-2 and lymphokine-activated killer cells. N Engl J Med 1988; 318(24): 1557–63.
23. Scalzo S, Gengaro A, Boccoli G, et al. Primary hypothyroidism associated with interleukin-2 and interferon alpha-2 therapy of melanoma and renal carcinoma. Eur J Cancer 1990; 26(11/12): 1152–6.
24. Atkins M, Mier J, Demchak P, et al. Thyroid dysfunction following IL-2 therapy. Proc ASCO 1990; 9: 186 (abstract # 720).
25. Pichert G, Jost LM, Zöbeli L, et al. Thyroiditis after treatment with interleukin-2 and interferon alpha-2a. Br J Cancer 1990; 62: 102–4.
26. Schwartzentruber DJ, White DE, Zweig MH, et al. Thyroid dysfunction associated with immunotherapy for patients with cancer. Cancer 1991; 68: 2384–90.
27. Jacobs EL, Clare-Salzler MJ, Chopra IJ, Figlin RA. Thyroid function abnormalities associated with the chronic outpatient administration of recombinant interleukin-2 and recombinant interferon-alpha. J Immunother 1991; 10: 448–55.
28. Ubhi SS, Horsburgh T, Veitch PS, Bell PRF. Anti-CD3 enhancement of cellular cytotoxicity in cancer patients treated with interleukin-2. Anticancer Res 1991; 11: 931–6.
29. Creaven PJ, Brenner DE, Cowens JW, et al. A phase I clinical trial of recombinant human tumor necrosis factor given daily for five days. Cancer Chemother Pharmacol 1989; 23: 186–91.
30. Silverman P, Berger NA. Recent clinical experience with tumor necrosis factor and advances in understanding its physiologic function and cellular activities. Curr Opinion Oncol 1990; 2: 1133–8.
31. Strieter RM, Remick DG, Ward PA, et al. Cellular and molecular regulation of tumor necrosis factor-alpha production by pentoxifylline. Biochem Biophys Res Commun 1988; 155(3): 1230–6.
32. Doherty GM, Jensen JC, Alexander HR, et al. Pentoxifylline suppression of tumor necrosis factor gene transcription. Surgery 1991; 110(2): 192–8.
33. Sampaio PE, Sarno EN, Galilly R, et al. Thalidomide selectively inhibits tumor necrosis factor alpha production by stimulated human monocytes. J Exp Med 1991; 173: 699–703.
34. Rosenberg SA, Lotze MT, Yang JC, et al. Experience with the use of high-dose interleukin-2

in the treatment of 652 cancer patients. Ann Surg 1989; 210: 474–85.
35. Parkinson DR, Abrams JS, Wiernik PH, et al. Interleukin-2 therapy in patients with metastatic malignant melanoma: A phase II study. J Clin Oncol 1990; 8(10): 1650–6.
36. Negrier S, Philip T, Stoter G, et al. Interleukin-2 with or without LAK cells in metastatic renal cell carcinoma: a report of a European multicenter study. Eur J Cancer Clin Oncol 1989; 25(Suppl 3): S21–8.
37. Mitchell MS, Kempf RA, Harel W, et al. Low-dose cyclophosphamide and low-dose interleukin-2 for malignant melanoma. Bull N Y Acad Med 1989; 65(1): 128–44.
38. McCabe MS, Stablein D, Hawkins MJ. The modified Group C experience – phase III randomized trials of IL-2 vs IL-2/LAK in advanced renal cell carcinoma and advanced melanoma. Proc ASCO 1991; 10: 213(abstract # 714).
39. Sleijfer D, Janssen R, Willemse P, et al. Subcutaneous (s.c.) interleukin-2 (IL-2) (Cetus) in patients (pts) with metastatic renal cell cancer (RCC). Proc ASCO 1991; 10: 163(abstract # 517).
40. Whitehead RP, Kopecky KJ, Samson MK, et al. Phase II study of intravenous bolus recombinant interleukin-2 in advanced malignant melanoma: Southwest Oncology Group Study. J Natl Cancer Inst 1991; 83: 1250–2.
41. Allison MAK, Jones SE, McGuffey P. Phase II trial of outpatient interleukin-2 in malignant lymphoma, chronic lymphocytic leukemia, and selected solid tumors. J Clin Oncol 1989; 7(1): 75–80.
42. Bukowski RM, Goodman P, Crawford ED, et al. Phase II trial of high-dose intermittent interleukin-2 in metastatic renal cell carcinoma: A Southwest Oncology Group Study. J Natl Cancer Inst 1990; 82(2): 143–6.
43. Klempner MS, Noring R, Mier JW, et al. An acquired chemotactic defect in neutrophils from patients receiving interleukin-2 immunotherapy. N Engl J Med 1990; 322(14): 959–65.
44. Snydman DR, Sullivan B, Gill M, et al. Nosocomial sepsis associated with interleukin-2. Ann Intern Med 1990; 112(2): 102–7.
45. Clark JW, Smith II JW, Steis RG, et al. Interleukin 2 and lymphokine-activated killer cell therapy: Analysis of a bolus interleukin-2 and continuous infusion interleukin-2 regimen. Cancer Res 1990; 50: 7343–50.
46. Dutcher JP, Gaynor ER, Boldt DH, et al. A phase II study of high-dose continuous infusion interleukin-2 with lymphokine-activated killer cells in patients with metastatic melanoma. J Clin Oncol 1991; 9(4): 641–8.
47. Sosman JA, Kohler PC, Hank JA, et al. Repetitive weekly cycles of interleukin-2. II. Clinical and immunologic effects of dose, schedule, and addition of indomethacin. J Natl Cancer Inst 1988; 80: 1451–61.
48. Thompson JA, Lee DJ, Lindgren CG, et al. Influence of dose and duration of infusion of interleukin-2 on toxicity and immunomodulation. J Clin Oncol 1988; 6: 669–78.
49. Gemlo BT, Palladino MA Jr, Jaffe HS, et al. Circulating cytokines in patients with metastatic cancer treated with recombinant interleukin 2 and lymphokine-activated killer cells. Cancer Res 1988; 48: 5864–7.
50. Richards JM, Bajorin DF, Vogelzang NJ, et al. Treatment of metastatic melanoma with continuous intravenous (CIV) IL2 ± LAK cells: A randomized trial. Proc ASCO 1990; 9: 279(abstract # 1080).
51. Stoter G, Fossa SD, Rugarli C, et al. Metastatic renal cell cancer treated with low-dose interleukin-2. A phase II multicenter study. Cancer Treat Rev 1989; 16: 111–3.
52. Parkinson DR. Lessons from the clinical trials of interleukin-2. Nat Immun Cell Growth Regul 1990; 9: 242–52.
53. Schall TJ, Bacon K, Toy KJ, Goeddel DV. Selective attraction of monocytes and T lymphocytes of the memory phenotype by RANTES. Nature 1990; 347: 669–71.
54. Hechtman DH, Cybulsky MI, Fuchs HJ, et al. Intravascular IL-8. Inhibitor of polymorphnuclear leukocyte accumulation at sites of acute inflammation. J Immunol 1991; 147(3): 883–92.

55. Huber AK, Kunkel SL, Todd RF III, Weiss SJ. Regulation of transendothelial neutrophil migration by endogenous interleukin-8. Science 1991; 254: 99–102.
56. Meyers FJ, Paradise C, Scudder SA, et al. A phase I study including pharmacokinetics of polyethylene glycol conjugated interleukin-2. Clin Pharmacol Ther 1991; 49(3): 307–13.
57. Urba WJ, Steis RG, Longo DL, et al. Immunomodulatory properties and toxicity of interleukin 2 in patients with cancer. Cancer Res 1990; 50: 185–92.
58. Whitehead RP, Ward D, Hemingway L, et al. Subcutaneous recombinant interleukin-2 in a dose escalating regimen in patients with metastatic renal cell adenocarcinoma. Cancer Res 1990; 50: 6708–15.
59. Sosman JA, Hank JA, Moore KH, et al. Prolonged Interleukin-2 (IL-2) treatment can augment immune activation without enhancing antitumor activity in renal cell carcinoma. Cancer Invest 1991; 9(1): 35–48.
60. Perez EA, Scudder SA, Meyers FA, et al. Weekly 24-hour continuous infusion interleukin-2 for metastatic melanoma and renal cell carcinoma: A phase I study. J Immunother 1991; 10: 57–62.
61. Creekmore SP, Harris JE, Ellis TM, et al. A phase I clinical trial of recombinant interleukin-2 by periodic 24-hour intravenous infusion. J Clin Oncol 1989; 7(2): 276–84.
62. West WH. Clinical application of continuous infusion of recombinant interleukin-2. Eur J Cancer Clin Oncol 1989; 25(Suppl 3): S11–S5.
63. Fortis C, Ferrero E, Biffi M, et al. Recombinant interleukin-2 and lymphokine-activated killer cells in renal cancer patients: II. characterization of cells cultured ex vivo and their contribution to the in vivo immunomodulation. Cancer Immunol Immunother 1991; 33: 128–32.
64. Pichert G, Jost LM, Fierz W, Stahel RA. Clinical and immune modulatory effects of alternative weekly interleukin-2 and interferon alpha-2a in patients with advanced renal cell carcinoma and melanoma. Br J Cancer 1991; 63: 287–92.
65. Denicoff KD, Durkin TM, Lotze MT, et al. The neuroendocrine effects of interleukin-2 treatment. J Clin Endocrin Metab 1989; 69(2): 402–10.
66. Hughes TK, Smith EM. Corticotropin (ACTH) induction of tumor necrosis factor alpha by monocytes. J Biol Regul Homeost Agents 1989; 3: 163–6.
67. Karalis K, Sano H, Redwine J, et al. Autocrine or paracrine inflammatory actions of corticotropin-releasing hormone in vivo. Science 1991; 254: 421–3.
68. Uchida A, Yanagawa E, Kokoschka EM, et al. In vitro modulation of human natural killer cell activity by interferon: generation of adherent suppressor cells. Br J Cancer 1984; 50: 483–92.
69. Thatcher N, Dazzi H, Johnson RJ, et al. Recombinant interleukin-2 (rIL-2) given intrasplenically and intravenously for advanced malignant melanoma. A phase I and II study. Br J Cancer 1989; 60: 770–4.
70. Gregorian SK, Battisto JR. Immunosuppression in murine renal cell carcinoma. I. Characterization of extent, severity and sources. Cancer Immunol Immunother 1990; 31: 325–34.
71. Gregorian SK, Battisto JR. Immunosuppression in murine renal cell carcinoma: II. Identification of responsible lymphoid cell phenotypes and examination of elimination of suppression. Cancer Immunol Immunother 1990; 31: 335–41.
72. Eisenthal A. Indomethacin up-regulates the generation of lymphokine-activated killer cell activity and antibody-dependent cellular cytotoxicity mediated by interleukin-2. Cancer Immunol Immunother 1990; 31(6): 342–8.
73. Wallick SC, Figari IS, Morris RA, et al. Immunoregulatory role of transforming growth factor beta (TGF-beta) in development of killer cells: comparison of active and latent TGF-beta$_1$. J Exp Med 1990; 172: 1777–84.
74. Kolitz JE, Wong GY, Welte K, et al. Phase I trial of recombinant interleukin-2 and cyclophosphamide: augmentation of cellular immunity and T-cell mitogenic response with long-term administration of rIL-2. J Biol Response Mod 1988; 7: 457–72.
75. Abrams JS, Rayner AA, Wiernik PH, et al. High-dose recombinant interleukin-2 alone: A regimen with limited activity in the treatment of advanced renal cell carcinoma. J Natl Cancer Inst 1990; 82(14): 1202–5.

76. Eisenhauer EA, Zee BC, Pater JL, Walsh WR. Trimetrexate: predictors of severe or life-threatening toxic effects. J Natl Cancer Inst 1988; 79: 1318–22.
77. Eisenthal A, Monselise J, Zinger R, Adler A. The effect of cimetidine on PBL from healthy donors and melanoma patients: augmentation of T cell responses to TCGF mitogens and alloantigens and of TCGF production. Cancer Immunol Immunother 1986; 21: 141–7.
78. Nair MPN, Schwartz SA. Effect of histamine and histamine antagonists on natural and antibody-dependent cellular cytotoxicity of human lymphocytes in vitro. Cell Immunol 1983; 81: 45–7.
79. Lindemann A, Hoeffken K, Schmidt RE, et al. A multicenter trial of interleukin-2 and low-dose cyclophosphamide in highly chemotherapy-resistant malignancies. Cancer Treat Rev 1989; 16 (Suppl A): 53–7.
80. Witherspoon RP, Lum LG, Storb R. Immunologic reconstitution after human marrow grafting. Semin Hematol 1984; 21(1): 2–10.
81. Atkinson K, Hansen JA, Storb R, et al. T-Cell subpopulations identified by monoclonal antibodies after human marrow transplantation. I. Helper-inducer and cytotoxic-suppressor subsets. Blood 1982; 59(6): 1292–8.
82. Ueda M, Harada M, Shiobara S, et al. T-lymphocyte reconstitution in long-term survivors after allogeneic and autologous marrow transplantation. Transplantation 1984; 37(6): 552–6.
83. Bosly A, Brice P, Humblet Y, et al. Interleukin-2 after autologous bone marrow transplantation as consolidative immunotherapy against minimal residual disease. Nouv Rev Fr Hematol 1990; 32: 13–16.
84. Syman M, Bosly A, Gisselbrecht C, et al. Immune reconstitution after bone-marrow transplantation. Cancer Treat Rev 1989; 16(Suppl A): 15–9.
85. Bosly AE, Staquet PJ, Doyen CM, et al. Recombinant human interleukin-2 restores in vitro T-cell colony formation by peripheral blood mononuclear cells after autologous bone marrow transplantation. Exp Hematol 1987; 15: 1048–54.
86. Heslop HE, Price GM, Prentice HG, et al. In vitro analysis of the interactions of recombinant IL-2 with regenerating lymphoid and myeloid cells after allogeneic marrow transplantation. J Immunol 1988; 140(10): 3461–6.
87. Heslop HE, Duncombre AS, Reittie JE, et al. Interleukin 2 infusion induces haematopoietic growth factors and modifies marrow regeneration after chemotherapy or autologous marrow transplantation. Br J Haematol 1991; 77: 237–44.
88. Heslop HE, Gottlieb DJ, Bianchi ACM, et al. In vitro induction of gamma interferon and tumor necrosis factor by interleukin-2 infusion following intensive chemotherapy or autologous marrow transplantation. Blood 1989; 74(4): 1374–80.
89. Higuchi CM, Thompson JA, Petersen FB, et al. Toxicity and immunomodulatory effects of interleukin-2 after autologous bone marrow transplantation for hematologic malignancies. Blood 1991; 77(12): 2561–8.
90. Soiffer R, Murray C, Cochran K, et al. Clinical and immunologic effects of prolonged continuous infusion of interleukin-2 (rIL-2) following allogeneic and autologous BMT. Proc ASCO 1991; 10: 211(abstract # 708).
91. Okaneya T, Ogawa A. Induction of cytotoxicity of the renal hilar lymph nodes by pedal subcutaneous administration of interleukin-2 in patients with renal cancer. Cancer 1991; 67: 1332–7.
92. Sarna G, Collins J, Figlin R, et al. A pilot study of intralymphatic interleukin-2. II. Clinical and biological effects. J Biol Response Mod 1990; 9: 81–6.
93. Shau H, Isacescu V, Ibayashi Y, et al. A pilot study of intralymphatic interleukin-2. II. Cytotoxic and surface marker changes of peripheral blood lymphocytes. J Biol Response Mod 1990; 9(1): 71–80.
94. Allegretta M, Atkins MB, Dempsey RA, et al. The development of anti-interleukin-2 antibodies in patients treated with recombinant human interleukin-2 (IL-2). J Clin Immunol 1986; 6(6): 481–90.
95. Yeilding N, Kirkwood J, Vlock D, et al. Preliminary analysis of a phase IB study of

intralymphatic and subcutaneous IL-2 in patients with local and regional metastasis in melanoma. Proc ASCO 1991; 10: 298(abstract # 1047).
96. Cortesina G, DeStefani A, Giovarelli M, et al. Treatment of recurrent squamous cell carcinoma of the head and neck with low doses of interleukin-2 injected perilymphatically. Cancer 1988; 62: 2482–5.
97. Cortesina G, DeStefani A, Galeazzi E, et al. Interleukin-2 injected around tumor-draining lymph nodes in head and neck cancer. Head Neck 1991; 13: 125–31.
98. Squadrelli-Saraceno M, Rivoltini L, Cantu G, et al. Local adoptive immunotherapy of advanced head and neck tumors with LAK cells and interleukin-2. Tumori 1990; 76: 566–71.
99. Lotze MT, Custer MC, Rosenberg SA. Intraperitoneal administration of interleukin-2 in patients with cancer. Arch Surg 1986; 121: 1373–9.
100. Beller U, Chachoua A, Speyer JL, et al. Phase IB study of low-dose intraperitoneal recombinant interleukin-2 in patients with refractory advanced ovarian cancer: rationale and preliminary report. Gynecol Oncol 1989; 34: 407–12.
101. Melioli G, Sertoli MR, Bruzzone M, et al. A phase I study of recombinant interleukin-2 intraperitoneal infusion in patients with neoplastic ascites: Toxic effects and immunologic results. Am J Clin Oncol 1991; 14(3): 231–7.
102. Roth A, Kirkwood JM. New clinical trials with interleukin-2: rationale for regional administration. Review. Nat Immun Cell Growth Regul 1989; 8: 153–64.
103. Thatcher N, Taylor P, Carroll KB, et al. Interleukin-2 in malignant pleural mesothelioma (and adenocarcinoma of the lung). The use of intrapleural and continuous intravenous infusions: preliminary results. Cancer Treat Rev 1989; 16(Suppl a): 161–2.
104. Eggermont AMM, Goey SH, Slingerland R, et al. Clinical and immunological evaluation of intrapleural (IPL) interleukin-2 (IL-2) in malignant pleural mesothelioma: a phase I-II study. Proc AACR 1991; 32: 206(abstract # 1228).
105. Klimberg IW, Pow-Sang JM, Cartwright CK, et al. Intravesical bacillus Calmette-Guerin for patients with high-risk superficial bladder cancer. Urology 1991; 37(2): 180–6.
106. Schwalb DM, Choudhury MS, Addonizio JC, et al. Maintenance intravesical bacillus Calmette-Guerin for superficial transitional carcinoma of the bladder: A retrospective study. Urology 1990; 36(3): 222–5.
107. Pizza GC, Severini G, Menniti D, et al. Tumor regression after intralesional injection of interleukin-2 (IL-2) in bladder cancer. Preliminary report. Int J Cancer 1984; 34(3): 359–67.
108. Huland E, Huland H. Local continuous high dose interleukin-2: A new therapeutic model for the treatment of advanced bladder carcinoma. Cancer Res 1989; 49: 5469–74.
109. Tubaro A, Velotti F, Stoppacciaro A, et al. Continuous intra-arterial administration of recombinant interleukin-2 in low-stage bladder cancer: A phase Ib study. Cancer 1991; 68(1): 56–61.
110. Velotti F, Stoppacciaro A, Ruco L, et al. Local activation of immune response in bladder cancer patients treated with intraarterial infusion of recombinant interleukin-2. Cancer Res 1991; 51: 2456–62.
111. Moser RP, Blacklock JB, Loudon WG, et al. Pilot study of intraventricular interleukin-2 for the treatment of leptomeningeal cancer. Proc ASCO 1991; 10: 129(abstract # 384).
112. Alberts DS, Kirkwood JM. Therapeutic modalities: Editorial overview. Curr Opinion Oncol 1990; 2: 1105–8.
113. Jost LM, Kirkwood JM. Immunotherapy of melanoma. In: Lejeune FJ, Chaudhuri PK, Das Gupta T, editors. Surgical Management of Malignant Melanoma. New York: Pergamon Press, 1991. In press.
114. McClay EF, Mastrangelo MJ, Bellet RE, Berd D. Combination chemotherapy and hormonal therapy in the treatment of malignant melanoma. Cancer Treat Rep 1987; 71: 465–9.
115. Atkins MB, Gould JA, Allegretta M, et al. Phase I evaluation of recombinant interleukin-2 in patients with advanced malignant disease. J Clin Oncol 1986; 4(9): 1380–91.
116. Kohler PC, Hank JA, Moore KH, et al. Phase I clinical trial of recombinant interleukin-2: a comparison of bolus and continuous intravenous infusion. Cancer Invest 1989; 7(3): 213–23.

117. Richards JM, Barker E, Latta J, et al. Phase I study of weekly 24-hour infusions of recombinant human interleukin-2. J Natl Cancer Inst 1988; 80: 1325–8.
118. Goldstein D, Sosman JA, Hank JA, et al. Repetitive weekly cycles of interleukin-2: Effect of outpatient treatment with a lower dose of interleukin 2 on non-major histocompatibility complex-restricted killer activity. Cancer Res 1989; 49: 6832–9.
119. Paciucci PA, Bhardwaj S, Odchimar R, et al. Immunotherapy for metastatic cancer with recombinant interleukin-2 (rIL2) by continuous infusion with and without adoptive cell transfer. Proc ASCO 1988; 7: 163(abstract # 630).
120. Poo W-j, Fynan T, Davis C, et al. High-dose recombinant interleukin-2 alone in patients with metastatic renal cell carcinoma. Proc ASCO 1991; 10: 173(abstract # 557).
121. Javapour N, Lalehzarian M. A phase I-II study of high-dose recombinant human interleukin-2 in disseminated renal-cell carcinoma. Semin Surg Oncol 1988; 4: 207–9.
122. West WH, Tauer KW, Yannelli JR, et al. Constant-infusion recombinant interleukin-2 in adoptive immunotherapy of advanced cancer. N Engl J Med 1987; 316(15): 898–905.
123. Boldt DH, Mills BJ, Gemlo BT, et al. Laboratory correlates of adoptive immunotherapy with recombinant interleukin-2 and lymphokine-activated killer cells in humans. Cancer Res 1988; 48: 4409–16.
124. Marth C, Gastl G, Zech J, et al. Characterization of an interferon-resistant mutant of the human breast cancer cell line BT-20. J Interferon Res 1987; 7: 195–202.
125. Mitchell MS, Kempf RA, Harel W, et al. Effectiveness and tolerability of low-dose cyclophosphamide and low-dose intravenous interleukin-2 disseminated melanoma. J Clin Oncol 1988; 6(3): 409–24.
126. Miyazaki A, Hanafusa T, Yamada K, et al. Predominance of T-lymphocytes in pancreatic islets and spleen of pre-diabetic non-obese diabetic (NOD) mice: A longitudinal study. Clin Exp Immunol 1985; 60: 622–30.
127. Blay JY, Combaret V, Negrier S, et al. IL1 and TNF concentrations as predictive factors of clinical response to IL2 in patients with renal cell carcinoma. Proc ASCO 1991; 10: 217(abstract # 732).
128. Hersey P, Coates A, Rallings M, et al. Comparative study on the effects of recombinant alpha-2 interferon on immune function in patients with disseminated melanoma. J Biol Response Mod 1986; 5: 236–49.
129. Cohen PJ, Lotze MT, Roberts JR, et al. The immunopathology of sequential tumor biopsies in patients treated with interleukin-2. Correlation of response with T-cell infiltration and HLA-DR expression. Am J Pathol 1987; 129(2): 208–16.

3. Interleukin-2 and lymphokine activated killer (LAK) cells

SYLVIE NEGRIER and THIERRY O. PHILIP

Historical rationale and laboratory aspects

Lymphokine-activated-killer cells are peripheral lymphocytes that develop, following exposure to Interleukin-2 (IL2), the ability to lyse tumour cells but not normal cells. This phenomenon has been extensively studied in the early eighties. These LAK cells appeared cytotoxic to non-cultured, natural killer-cell-resistant tumour cells without antigenic stimulation implicating killing in a non MHC-restricted manner [1, 2]. Extensive studies of the precursors of LAK cells have revealed that they are constituted in part of activated cytotoxic T cells but consist predominantly of activated Natural-Killer (NK) cells [3, 4].

After these first in vitro experimental studies, LAK cells were generated and transferred into mice bearing pulmonary and hepatic metastases from a wide variety of established tumours (e.g. melanomas, sarcomas, colon or bladder carcinomas) [5–7]. The injection of these cells along with the systemic administration of IL2 induced significant tumour regressions. In most experiments the administration of IL2 in combination with LAK-cells appeared necessary to induce these tumour regressions [8]. Systemic IL2 alone was, however, able to generate LAK-cells in vivo and tumour regressions in animal tumour models were dependent on the dose of IL2. Since they represented potential therapeutic tools for cancer patients, these techniques were tested in humans.

During the first phase of this approach, therapy with LAK-cells was proven to be feasible [8, 9]. Patients tolerated injections of up to 2×10^{11} LAK-Cells with acceptable toxicity. Concurrently, different phase I studies using a variety of schedules of intravenous IL2 were conducted to determine the maximal tolerated doses. No tumour regression was observed in any of these patients. Conversely, when the combination of IL2 together with LAK-cells was applied in patients with advanced cancer, significant tumour regressions were noted in several patients [8, 10].

Since IL2 combined with LAK cells appeared more efficient than IL2 alone, most initial phase II studies were performed using this combination.

From a practical point of view, LAK-cell development for therapeutic use

J. Wagstaff (ed.), The Role of Interleukin-2 in the Treatment of Cancer Patients, 29-43.

was rather complex, costly and time consuming. The initial report of large-scale production of LAK-cells for use in adoptive immunotherapy appeared in 1986 [11]. LAK-cell precursors [10^9 to 10^{11} cells) were obtained by repeated leukophereses. These procedures were done 1 to 2 days after cessation of IL2 administration since this date corresponds to the IL2 induced rebound lymphocytosis. The mononuclear cells obtained from leukophereses were initially purified with Fycoll-hypaque gradients. These procedures were simplified with the use of an automated blood cell separator [12]. Furthermore, it was shown that the non purified cell cultures improved mononuclear cell recovery as well as LAK-cell activation [13, 14].

Several further improvements occurred in harvest, culture and collection before reinjection of these cells. These new procedures reduce the frequency of handling of large volumes of cell culture material. Some modifications such as the replacement of the pooled human AB serum with 2 % heat inactivated autologous plasma appeared safe and costed less [13]. More recently, cultures have been successfully developed in serum-free-medium [15, 16].

Some investigators developed efforts in purifying LAK precursors before initiation of the IL2 cultures [17, 18]. Using the adherence properties of LAK precursors to plastic, these authors generated adherent-purified-LAK-Cells (A-LAK) which appeared significantly more active in terms of proliferation as well as cytotoxicity than conventional LAK-cells.

More recently, the production of a different purified population of cells called Lymphokine Activated Natural Killer cells (LANAK) was reported [19]. In vitro, these LANAK appeared 100 times more efficient than their autologous LAK counterparts.

The mechanisms of action of LAK-cells are not completely understood. In patients receiving IL2 and LAK-cells, dense lymphoïd infiltrates can be seen within tumour lesions and LAK-cells have been proven to divide in vivo, in animals receiving IL2 [20, 21]. However, no clinical data are consistent with the fact that LAK-cells traffic specifically to tumour sites [21]. The antitumour effect of LAK-cells can be related to the direct cytotoxicity of these cells or to antibody-dependent cellular cytotoxicity (ADCC). The in vivo production of cytokines by LAK-cells as well as autologous cells activated by IL2 is more likely to play an important role in the tumour regression phenomenon [22–24].

More specific effector cells than LAK-cells are still being actively searched for and tested i.e. Activated Killer Monocytes (AKM), tumour infiltrating lymphocytes (TIL) [25, 26]. Nevertheless, LAK cells were the first large-scale cultured cells that could be successfully administered as a therapeutic tool and as such, they represent the first step towards effective adoptive cellular therapy in cancer patients.

IL2 regimens used in combination with LAK cells

Systemic administration

IL2 and LAK cell protocols were initiated in the NCI Surgery Branch using high intravenous bolus doses of IL2 [8, 10]. In these studies, patients received IL2 by intravenous bolus infusion every 8 hours, usually at a dose of 600 000 IU/kg for 5 days. The daily dose of IL2 in this protocol is approximately 50 $\times$ 10^6 IU/m^2.

The schedule of administration is shown on Figure 1.

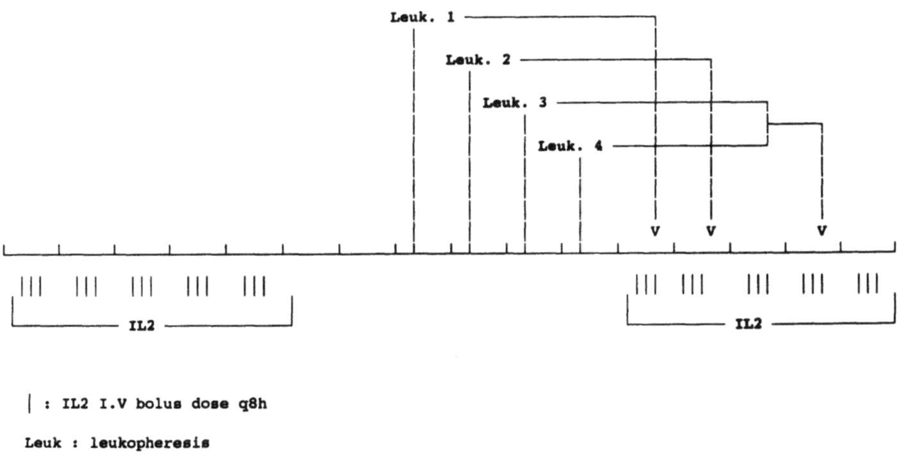

Figure 1. Scheme of one course of IL2 plus LAK cells according to Rosenberg's schedule [10].

Some authors reproduced Rosenberg's schedule in different types of tumour, but the toxicity of this treatment has deterred others [27, 28]. A different regimen was therefore tested. The first report of continuous infusion of IL2 together with LAK cells was made by West et al. in 1987 [28]. The continuous infusion regimen utilises lower daily doses than with bolus administration, i.e. 18 $\times$ 10^6 IU/m^2/day. The duration is identical to that of Rosenberg's regimen with only the dose and the mode of administration being different.

LAK cell administration is also possible together with a combined therapy of IL2 and Interferon alpha [29]. The administration of IL2 and LAK cells can also be used in paediatric oncology [30].

The results reported by different authors using systemic IL2 and LAK cells are summarised in Table 1. According to the data provided by these authors, we calculated that the mean amount of reinjected LAK cells was 4.8 $\times$ 10^{10} per course (range 0.5 to 10.1 $\times$ 10^{10}).

Table 1. Main results reported in the literature on the use of intravenous IL2 together with LAK cells

Authors	IL2 schedule and dose	Diagnosis	Number of patients	CR	PR	CR + PR (%)
Rosenberg et al. [10]	720 000 IU/kg q8 h	Renal	72	8	17	35
		Melanoma	48	4	6	21
		Colorectal	30	1	4	17
		NHL	7	1	3	–
		Sarcoma	6	0	0	–
		Lung	5	0	0	–
		Other	10	0	0	–
Schoof et al. [31]	30 000 U/kg q8 h	Renal	10	1	4	–
		Melanoma	9	1	4	–
		Lymphoma	3	1	1	–
		Colorectal	4	0	0	–
		Ovarian	1	1	0	–
		Sarcoma	1	0	0	–
Dutcher et al. [32]	100 000 U/kg q8 h	Melanoma	32	1	5	19
Thompson et al. [33]	1×10^6 U/m^2 q8 h	Melanoma	4	0	0	–
		Renal	3	0	0	–
		Colorectal	4	0	0	–
	3×10^6 U/m^2/d	Melanoma	4	0	0	–
		Renal	8	1	0	–
		Colorectal	1	0	0	–
West et al. [28]	16.7×10^6 UI/m^2/d CI	Melanoma	10	0	5	–
		Renal	6	0	3	–
		Lung	5	0	1	–
		Breast	1	0	0	–
		Lymphoma	2	0	2	–
		Colon	13	0	0	0
Paciucci et al. [34]	1–5 $\times 10^6$IU/m^2/d CI	Melanoma	5	0	1	–
		Renal	9	0	1	–
		Lymphoma	4	0	1	–
		CML	3	0	0	–
		Sarcoma	2	0	1	–
		Colorectal	1	0	1	–
Negrier et al. [35]	18×10^6 IU/m^2/d CI	Renal	51	5	9	27
Stahel et al. [36]	30 000 U/kg q8 h	Renal	14	5	9	21
		Melanoma	7	0	3	–
		Colon	2	0	0	–

Table 1. Continued

Authors	IL2 schedule and dose	Diagnosis	Number of patients	CR	PR	CR + PR (%)
Hawkins [37]	100 000 U/kg q8 h	Renal	32	2	3	16
		Melanoma	32	1	5	19
		Colorectal	19	1	2	16
Parkinson et al. [38]	600 000 IU/kg q8h + 18×10^6 IU/m²/d CI	Renal	47	2	2	9
Bar et al. [39]	6000 IU/kg q8h + 18×10^6 IU/m²/d CI	Melanoma	50	1	6	14
Dutcher et al. [40]	18×10^6 IU/m²/d CI	Melanoma	33	0	1	3
Philip et al. [29]	24×10^6 IU/m² 98 h IFNα 5×10^6 IU/m² q8 h	Renal	34	2	6	24
Negrier et al. [30]	18×10^6 IU/m²/d CI	Neuroblastoma	15	0	0	0
Dillman et al. [41]		Melanoma	29	2	2	14
		Renal	23	0	1	4
		Lymphoma	6	0	0	–
		Colon	6	0	0	–
		Sarcoma	3	0	0	–
		Ovarian	3	0	0	–
		Other	22	2*	1*	3
Margolin et al. [42]	600 000 IU/kg q8h + 18×10^6IU/ m²/d CI	Lymphoma	27	0	2	7

The percentage of response is calculated only when the total number of patients in each series is > 10

* 2 CR in lung carcinoma and in appendix carcinoma, 1 PR in thyroid carcinoma

The overall response rates obtained through those series in each tumour type are shown in Table 2.

Although, with small numbers of patients, some histological types of cancer have been treated. Renal adenocarcinoma and melanoma obviously appear as the most sensitive tumours to IL2 therapy. In addition, the best complete response rate is achieved in metastatic renal cell cancer. Figures 2 and 3 show examples of complete remission in patients with metastatic renal cancer and melanoma. Although all the authors do not list the sites of tumour regression in detail, responses have been noted at a variety of sites. In melanoma and renal

Table 2. Overall response rates drawn from the different studies reported in each tumour type

Tumour type	Number of patients	CR	PR	CR + PR (%)
Melanoma	253	10	33	36 [17]
Renal	309	26	52	78 [25]
Colorectal	67	1	7	9 [13]
Lymphoma	49	2	9	11 [22]
Sarcoma	12	0	1	1 [8]

CR: complete response, PR: partial response

carcinoma, lymph nodes, cutaneous and subcutaneous tissues represent the most common sites of response, whilst liver, bone and kidney lesions have also been reported to respond. [10, 28, 32].

We calculated the median duration of response from the data that were available for review. Median duration of partial response is 6 months (range 1 to 43+) and median duration of complete response is 23 months (range 6 to 63+).

Very few data regarding the survival of these patients are available. Rosenberg et al. [21] reported a median survival of 20 months in their cohort of patients treated with IL2 + LAK cells. The interim analysis of European studies in metastatic renal cell carcinoma indicate a median survival of 1 year in patients receiving IL2 + LAK cells, but the median follow up has not been reached yet [35]. The toxicity of treatments with LAK cells and IL2 is comparable to that observed with the administration of intravenous IL2 alone. For example, toxic events observed in 2 cohorts of patients receiving LAK cells are shown in Table 3.

In our own experience, we have noted that LAK cell reinjections were commonly followed by an increase of the usual toxic signs of IL2, i.e. fever, chills, malaise and hypotension. LAK cells were, however, involved in one toxic death observed in a child with advanced neuroblastoma [30]. In this 21 kg child, a large number of LAK cells (e.g. 9.2×10^{10} cells) were reinjected, leading to interstitial lung infiltrates and respiratory distress.

Regional administration of LAK cells

Since no clinical study has demonstrated that LAK cells return to tumour sites after reinjection, several attempts have been made to administer LAK cells locally.

Several authors have reported the instillation of LAK cells directly at the site of brain tumours, as well as intrathecal injections in cases of meningeal carcinomatosis [43–48]. A survey of the different attempts to treat brain tumours with LAK cells showed that tumour lesions were not easily measurable and that, in some cases, LAK cell therapy was performed just after surgical resection [43–47]. In these conditions, the most consistent results have to be drawn from the survival follow-up of the patients. Nevertheless, some tumour

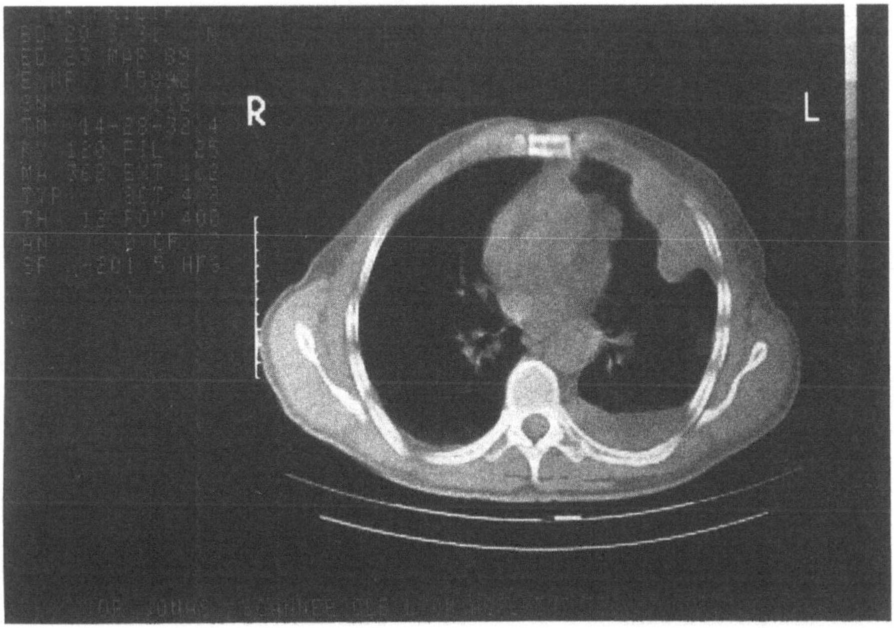

A

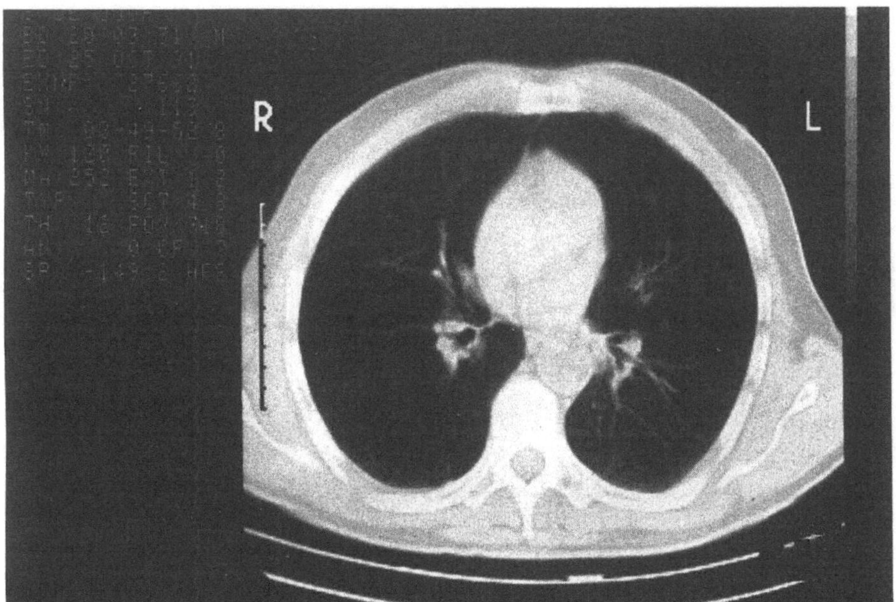

B

Figure 2. Example (CT scan) of a persistant complete remission (2 years +) in a patient with pleural, pericardial and rib metastases of renal adenocarcinoma.

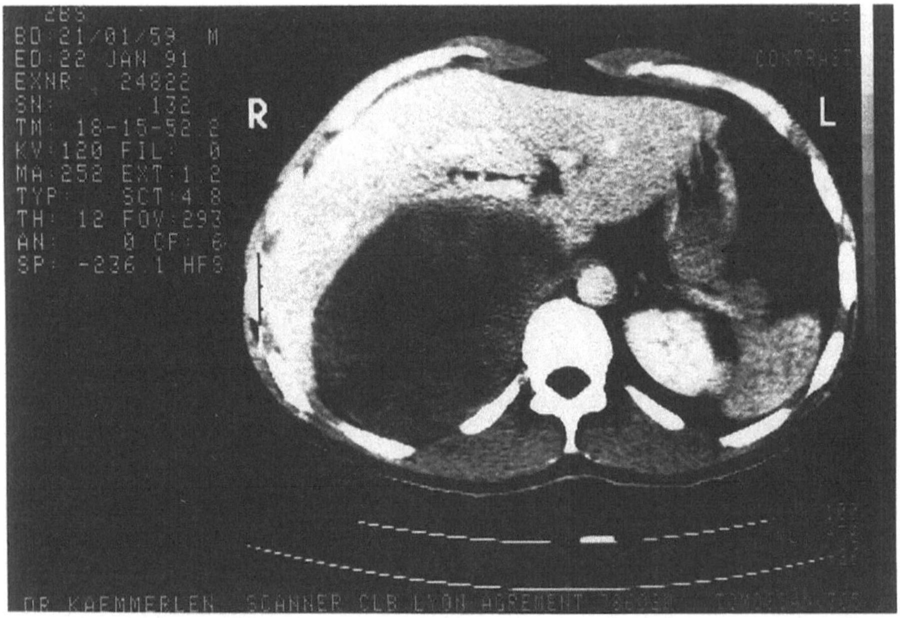

A

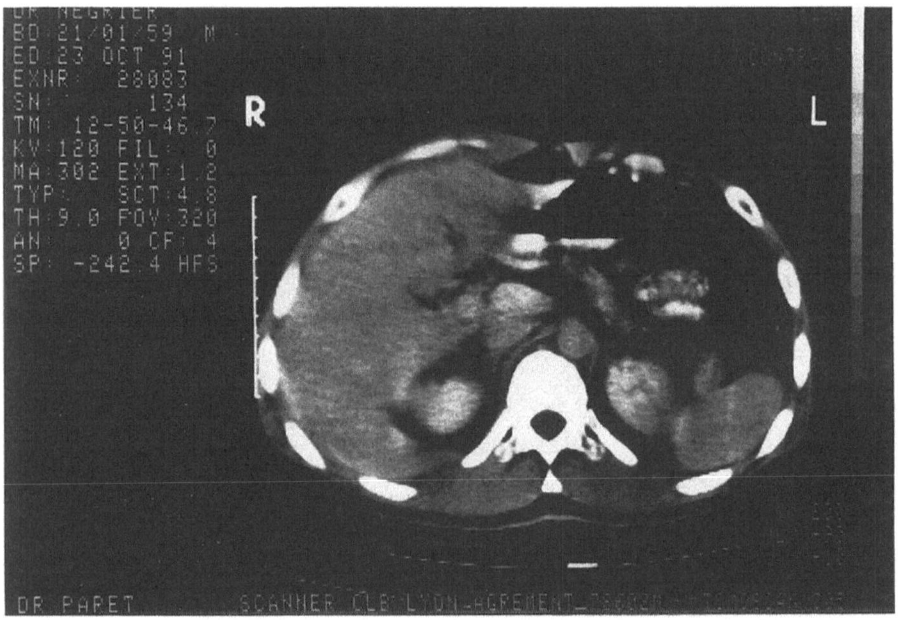

B

Figure 3. Example (CT scan) of a persistent complete remission (10 months +) in a patient with adrenal metastases of melanoma.

Table 3. Clinical toxicities observed during immunotherapy with LAK cells in patients with metastatic renal cell carcinoma [29]

Side effects	Incidence	
	IL2 + LAK n = 22	IL2 + IFN + LAK n = 34
Fever	100%	100%
Erythema	86%	100%
Diarrheoa	68%	90%
Hypotension*	50%	84%
Pruritus	63%	78%
Sommnolence	59%	71%
Weight gain	72%	63%
5 to 10%	54%	50%
> 10%	18%	9%
Oliguria	59%	53%
Tachycardia	22%	53%
Stomatitis	9%	53%
Vomiting	68%	50%
Dyspnoea	36%	37%
Acute renal failure**	36%	28%
Alopecia	18%	21%
Diffuse cyanosis	13%	18%
Thoracic pains	13%	16%
Assisted ventilation	9%	3%
Coma	4%	3%
Toxic death	0%	3%
Sepsis	4%	0%

* Hypotension requiring pressor agents.
** Creatinine > 400 μmol/l.

regressions were achieved in 7 of the 32 patients with an evaluable tumour [44–47]. The interest of these studies is obvious in diseases for which conventional therapies are inadequate.

Some significant tumour regressions have been also reported using LAK cell infusion into the peritoneal cavity. Furthermore, some experiments demonstrated that LAK activity was maintained in the peritoneal cavity and systemic toxicity was reduced [49, 50].

Intrapleural instillation of IL2 and LAK-cells was also performed, leading to the disappearance of malignant cells in 9 of 11 patients [51]. Some tumour responses have also been reported with the injection of IL2 and LAK-cells into the lymphatic vessels of patients with different types of advanced cancer [52].

The toxicity of LAK cells administered regionally was not specific except in case of brain tumours. Indeed, authors observed the common induction of an increased intracranial hypertension syndrome.

Although some of these approaches gave interesting results, they remain however, experimental techniques.

Use of LAK cells in cancer patients

As proven by the available data concerning their therapeutic use LAK-cells have been extensively used and studied during the past 8 years. However, from a clinical point of view, several still debatable points are apparent.

IL2 + LAK: response rates and their variations

The concept of immunotherapy in oncology was raised again in the late seventies; but it became a reality in 1984 when treatments combining recombinant IL2 and LAK cells were successfully performed in patients with advanced cancer.

Tumour regressions, sometimes complete and achieved in patients with widespread diseases indicated that another way to treat cancer patients was possible. As shown in the literature, IL2 together with LAK cells was applied in different institutions and different countries, and the results from Rosenberg et al. [8] were reproduced, though sometimes with lower response rates. The differences in the number of responding patients can be due to at least 2 different reasons. In metastatic renal cell cancer, the selection of patients seems to be the most important factor.

As acknowledged by Rosenberg himself [21], patients accrued into the IL2 + LAK cell trials at the National Cancer Institute had a lower tumour burden than those treated with the same protocol schedules in the 6 institutions of the IL2/LAK Extra Mural Working Group [37]. Therefore, the response rate of IL2 + LAK cell treatments in renal cell cancer patients is more likely to average 25 or 30%.

In melanoma patients, though patient selection can also interfere, results appeared more alike when identical schedules and doses of treatment were used. Response rates obtained with high bolus doses of IL2 together with LAK cells are around 20%, and the number of complete responses obtained in this disease is smaller than that obtained in renal carcinoma, i.e. 4% vs. 9% respectively. In addition, the dose of IL2 administered to the patient appears to be an important factor for the efficacy of the treatment in melanoma.

The most conspicuous example was given by Dutcher et al. [32, 40] in 2 successive cohorts of patients with metastatic melanoma. Even though these studies were not carried out as prospective randomized trials, the 2 populations were virtually identical when usual prognosis factors were compared, i.e. bulk of the disease, number of tumour sites, percentage of soft tissue lesions only, and performance status. Bolus doses of IL2 together with LAK cells yielded a 19% response rate versus 3% with continuous IL2 infusion and LAK cells.

In addition to differences in the schedule of administration, we must note that the doses of IL2 were quite different, i.e. around 54×10^6 IU/m^2/day with bolus doses versus 18×10^6 IU/m^2/day with continuous infusion. We think that the difference in response rates is most likely to be related to the dose-effect of IL2.

IL2 + LAK: activity versus tumour type

Since in early trials conducted in the NCI patients with renal cell cancer and melanoma showed the most significant anticancer responses, the majority of patients further selected for treatment with IL2 and LAK cells suffered from these two types of tumours. This new therapeutic approach was encouraging since renal cell cancer is known to be resistant to conventional chemotherapy, and melanoma is only sensitive to very few cytotoxic drugs.

In other tumour types, results must be interpreted quite prudently. First of all, no formal phase II trial using IL2 + LAK cells has been conducted yet in these patients. The available data come from broad phase II studies, which raises again the problem of patient selection. Results of different studies using varying schedules and doses of IL2 are summarized in Table 2. Some remarks can, however, be made upon these results.

IL2 + LAK does not appear efficacious in metastatic sarcoma but seems to have some degree of activity in metastatic colorectal cancer. A survey of the literature on the most recently evaluated agents given as monotherapy for colorectal cancer treatment shows that IL2 + LAK comes second after 5 Fluorouracil [53]. This means that a combination of IL2 and 5FU could be of interest; several studies are ongoing in an attempt to evaluate this combined therapy.

In lymphoma, IL2 + LAK has indeed some efficacy. The problem in this particular disease is now to determine the optimal place of IL2 therapy within the complex chemotherapy regimens that are an integral part of the treatment of lymphoma.

IL2 and LAK cells were merely evaluated, in the recent past years, as monotherapy regimens; IL2, however, could be interesting to test in a different approach. IL2 is effectively a potential biological response modifier but was until now as such under-investigated. Some encouraging results, mainly obtained with the combination of IL2 and cisplatinum, argue for the development of clinical trials in this setting [54, 55].

LAK Cells: therapeutic benefit?

Regarding the combination of IL2 and LAK cells, all investigators involved in immunotherapy programs wondered whether LAK cells were really necessary. LAK cells were used in humans because of the results obtained in vitro and in animal experiments [5, 7]. They appeared indeed as the major effector of IL2 anticancer activity in vitro; and the most significant tumour regressions noted in animal models were achieved through the administration of IL2 together with LAK cells. But LAK cell development for therapeutic use requires time, technical work and financial cost. In our institute, the cost of LAK cell development for one single patient has been evaluated at about 7300 US$.

Tumour regressions were also achieved with IL2 alone and the response rates were not significantly different from those obtained with LAK cells.

In the European studies conducted in patients with metastatic renal cell cancer, though these were not randomized, the best response rate was obtained with IL2 + LAK cells, i.e. 27% vs. 19% for IL2 alone [35]. This difference, which is not statistically significant, and was mostly related to the difference in IL2 doses delivered in each cohort of patients.

The NCI Surgery Branch conducted a prospective randomized trial in 181 patients with advanced cancer [56]. The overall response rates were comparable, i.e. 28% (LAK/IL2) vs. 20% (IL2), although the incidence of complete responses tended to be higher in the arm with IL2 + LAK cells.

As far as a randomized phase II trial with response rates under 30% can be trusted, the conclusion to be drawn is that LAK cells are not necessary. But since the mechanisms of anticancer activity in patients receiving LAK cells and IL2 are not clearly understood, LAK cells cannot be considered as useless.

Practically, the development of LAK cells has been dropped by most centres because of its expensiveness and the lack of a substantial benefit for the patients.

Conclusions

IL2 with LAK cells represent the first large scale and reproducible application of adoptive immunotherapy in humans. After the meaningful preclinical work that has been done, IL2 and LAK cells have been used in therapeutic trials in numerous countries giving substantial results. At this point of time, the mechanisms of action of LAK cells in vivo are not yet completely understood. Even if the transfer of LAK cells together with IL2 administration seems slightly more efficient than the use of IL2 alone, the rationale for the development of these cells remains questionable.

Therefore, a variety of experiments have been and are still being conducted in order to improve the clinical results of immunotherapy. The most remarkable were, in our opinion, the use of ambulatory immunotherapy regimens and the development of IL2 activated TIL (Tumour Infiltrating Lymphocytes) [26, 57]. In addition to their own therapeutic potential, TIL were also more recently developed for gene transfer experiments [58]. These innovative techniques applied in humans have opened a new field of medical treatment using gene-modified cells as a therapeutic tool.

LAK cell development remains, however, an important step in the pioneering work of the immunotherapy of cancer.

References

1. Grimm EA, Mazumder A, Zhang HZ, Rosenberg SA. Lymphokine activated killer cell phenomenom. J Exp Med 1982; 155: 1823–41.
2. Rosenstein M, Yron I, Kaufmann Y, Rosenberg SA Lymphocyte activated killer cells: lysis of

fresh syngeneic natural killer-resistant murine tumor cells by lymphocytes cultured in Interleukin 2. Cancer Res 1984; 44: 1946–53
3. Grimm EA, Ramsey KM, Mazumder A, et al. Lymphokine-activated killer cell phenomenom. II Precursor phenotype is biologically distinct from peripheral T. lymphocytes, memory cytotoxic thymus-derived lymphocytes, and natural killer cells. J Exp Med 1983; 157: 884–97.
4. Philips JH, Lanier LL. Dissection of the lymphokine-activated killer phenomenom. Relative contribution of peripheral bolld natural killer cells and T. lymphocytes to cytolysis. J Exp Med 1986; 164: 814–23.
5. Mazumder A, Rosenberg SA. Successful immunotherapy of naturel killer-resistant established pulmonary melanome metastases by the intravenous adoptive transfer of syngeneic lymphocytes activated in vitro by Interleukin 2. J Exp Med 1984; 159: 495–507.
6. Mule JJ, Shu S, Schwarz SL, Rosenberg SA. Adoptive immunotherapy of established pulmonary metastases with LAK-cells and recombinant Interleukin-2. Science 1984; 225: 1487–9.
7. Lafreniere R, Rosenberg SA. Successful immunotherapy of murine experimental hepatic metastases with lymphokine-activated killer cells and recombinant Interleukin-2. Cancer Res 1985; 45: 3735–41.
8. Rosenberg SA, Lotze MT, Muul LM, et al. Observations on the systemic administration of autologous lymphokine-activated killer cells and recombinant INterleukin-2 to patients with metastatic cancer. N Engl J Med 1985; 313: 1485–92.
9. Rosenberg SA. Immunotherapy of cancer by systemic administration of lymphoïd cells plus Interleukin-2. J Biol Response Modif 1984; 3: 501–11.
10. Rosenberg SA, Lotze MT, Muul LM, et al. A progress report on the treatment of 157 patients with advanced cancer using lymphokine activated killer cells and Interleukin-2 or high dose Interleukin-2 alone. N Engl J Med 1987; 316: 889–905.
11. Muul LM, Director EP, Hyatt C, Rosenberg SA. Large-scale production of hyman lymphokine-activated killer cells for use in adoptive immunotherapy. J Immunol Methods 1986; 88: 265–72.
12. Muul LM, Nason-burchenal K, Carter CS, et al. Development of an automated closed system for generation of human lymphokine-activated killer (LAK) cells for use in adoptive immnotherapy. J Immunol Methods 1987; 101: 171–81.
13. Favrot MC, Coze C, Combaret V, et al. Lymphokine-activated killer cell expansion of the culture technique. Mol Biother 1990; 2: 32–37
14. Yanelli JR, Thurman GB, Dickerson SG, et al. An improved method for the generation of human lymphokine activated killer cells. J Immunol Methods 1987; 100: 137–45.
15. Jadus MR, Thurman GB, Mrowea-Bastin A, Yannelli JR. The generation of human lymphokine activated-killer cells in various serum free-media. J Immunol Methods 1988; 109: 169–74.
16. Muul LM, Nason-Burchenal K, Hyatt C, Schwarz J, Slavin S, Director EP, Rosenberg SA. Studies of serum-free culture medium in the generation of kymphokine-activated killer cells. J Immunol Methods 1987; 105: 183–92.
17. Whiteside TL, Wang YL, Selker RG, Herberman RB. In vitro generation and antitumor activity of adherant lymphokine-activated killer cells froml the blood of patients with brain tumors. Cancer Res 1988; 48: 6069, 6075.
18. Melder RJ, Whiteside TL, Vujancovic NL, et al. Human adherant lymphokine-activated killer cells (A-LAK). A new approach to generating anti-tumor effects for adoptive immunotherapy. Cancer Res 1988; 48: 3461–68.
19. Hercend T, Farace F, Baume D, et al. Immunotherapy with lymphokine-activated natural killer cells and recombinant Interleukin-2: A feasability trial in metastatic renal cell carcinoma. J Biol Response Modif 1990; 9: 546–55.
20. Ettinghausen SE, Lipford EH, Mule JJ, et al. Recombinant Interleukin-2 stimulates invivo proliferation of adoptively transfered lymphokine-activated killer (LAK) cells. J Immunol 1985; 135: 3623–35.

21. Yang JC, Rosenberg SA. Adoptive cellular therapy: preclinical studies in biological therapy of cancer. In De Vita, Hellman, Rosenberg (eds.). JB Lippincott Company, 1991: 197–213.
22. Lotze MT, Matory YL, Ettinghausen SE, et al. In vivo administration of purified human Interleukin-2. Half life and immunologic effects and expansion of peripheral lymphoid cells in vivo with recombinant IL-2. J Immunol 1985; 135: 2865–74.
23. Gemlo BT, Palladino MA, Jaffe HS, et al. Circulating cytokines in patients with metastatic cancer treated with recombinant Interleukin-2 and lymphokine-activated killer cells. Cancer Res 1988; 48: 5864–72.
24. Blay JY, Favrot MC, Negrier S, et al. Correlation between clinical response to Interleukin-2 therapy and substained production of tumor necrosis factor. Cancer Res 1990; 50: 2371–4.
25. Yanelli JR, Stevenson GW, Stevenson HC. Cancer adoptive cellular immunotherapy. In: Principles of cancer biotherapy. Eds. Oldham Dekker, Inc. N.Y, 1991: 503–23.
26. Rosenberg SA, Packard BS, Aebersold PM, et al. Use of tumor infiltrating lymphocytes and Interleukin-2 in the immunotherapy of patients with metastatic melanoma, special report. N Engl J Med 1988; 319: 1976–80.
27. Moertel CG. On lymphokines, cytokines and breakthroughs. J Am Med Assoc 1986; 256: 3141–8.
28. West WH, Tauer KW, Yanneli JR, et al. Constant infusion recombinant interleukin-2 in adoptive immunotherapy of advanced cancer. N Engl J Med 1987; 316 (15): 898–905.
29. Philip T, Negrier S, Mercatello A, et al. Interleukin-2 in the treatment of metastatic renal cell cancer: 77 patients treated in Lyon. In Gardiner (ed). Insights into Immunotherapy. London: Caldwell, 1990: 23–30.
30. Negrier S, Michon J, Floret D, et al. Interleukin-2 and lymphokine-activated killer cells in 15 children with advanced metastatic neuroblastoma. J Clin Oncol 1991; 9: 1363–70.
31. Schoof DD, Gramolini BA, Davidson DL, et al. Adoptive immunotherapy of humain cancer using low-dose recombinant interleukin-2 and lymphokine-activated killer cells. Cancer Res 1988; 48: 5007–10.
32. Dutcher JP, Creekmore S, Weiss GR, et al. A phase II study of interleukin-2 and lymphokine-activated killer cells in patients with metastatic malignant melanoma. J Clin Oncol 1989; 7: 477–85.
33. Thompson JA, Lee DJ, Lindgren CG, et al. Influence of schedule of interleukin-2 administration on therapy with interleukin-2 and lymphokine-activated killer cells. Cancer Res 1989; 49: 235–40.
34. Paciucci PA, Holland JF, Glidewell, et al. Recombinant interleukin-2 continuous infusion and adoptive transfer of recombinant interleukin-2 activated cells in patients with advanced cancer. J Clin Oncol 1989; 7: 869–78.
35. Negrier S, Philip T, Stoter G, et al. Interleukin-2 with or without LAK cells in metastatic renal cell carcinoma: a report of a european multicentre study. Eur J Cancer Clin Oncol 1989; 25: S21–S28.
36. Stahel RA, Sculier J, Jost LM, et al. Tolerance and effectiveness of recombinant interleukin-2 (r-met Hu IL2 (ala 125)) and lymphokine-activated killer cells in patients with metastatic solid tumours. Eur J Cancer Clin Oncol 1989; 25: 965–72.
37. Hawkins MJ. PPO Updates IL-2/LAK. Princ Oncol 1989; 3: 1–14.
38. Parkinson DR, Fischer RI, Rayner AA, et al. Therapy of renal cell carcinoma with interleukin-2 and lymphokine-activated killer cells: phase II experience with a hybrid bolus and continuous infusion interleukin-2 regimen. J Clin Oncol 1990; 8: 1630–6.
39. Bar MH, Sznol M, Atkins MB, et al. Metastatic malignant melanoma treated with combined bolus and continuous infusion interleukin-2 and lymphokine-activated killer cells. J Clin Oncol 1990; 8: 1138–47.
40. Dutcher JP, Gaynor ER, Boldt DH, et al. A phase II study of high dose continuous infusion interleukin-2 with lymphokines-activated killer cells: not the optimal schedule for metastatic melanoma. J Clin Oncol 1991; 9: 641–8.
41. Dillman RO, Oldham RK, Tauer KW, et al. Continuous interleukin-2 and lymphokine-

activated killer cells for advanced cancer: a national biotherapy study group trial. J Clin Oncol 1991; 9: 1233–40.
42. Margolin KM, Aronson FR, Sznol M, et al. Phase II trial of high dose interleukin-2 and lymphokine-activated killer cells in Hodgkin's disease and non Hodgkin's lymphoma J Immunother 1991; 10: 214–20.
43. Jacobs SK, Wilson DJ, Kornblith PL, et al. Interleukin-2 or autologous lymphokine-activated killer cell treatment of malignant glioma: phase I trial. Cancer Res 1986: 46: 2101–4.
44. Yoshida S, Tanaka R, Takai N, et al. Local administration of autologous lymphokine-activated killer cell and recombinant interleukin-2 to patients with malignant brain tumors. Cancer Res 1988; 48: 5011–6.
45. Ingram M, Jacques S, Freshwater DB, et al. Salvage immunotherapy of malignant glioma. Arch Surg 1987; 122: 1483–6.
46. Merchant RE, Merchant LH, Cook SHS, et al. Intralesional infusion of lymphokineactivated killer (LAK) cells and recombinant interleukin-2 (rIL2) for the treatment of patients withmalignant brain tumor. Neurosurgery 1988; 23: 725–32.
47. Barba D, Saris SC, Holder C, et al. Immunotherapy of humain glial tumors: report of multiples dose intratumoral infusions of lymphokine-activated killer cells and interleukin-2. J Neurosurg 1988; 70: 175–82.
48. Himizu K, Okamoto Y, Miyato Y, et al. Adoptive immunotherapy of humain meningeal gliomatosis and carcinomatosis with LAK cells and recombinant interleukin-2. J Neurosurg 1987; 66: 519–21.
49. Lotze MT, Custer MC, Rosenberg SA Intraperitoneal administration of interleukin-2 in patients with cancer. Arch Surg 1986; 121: 1373.
50. Urba WJ, Clark JW, Steis RG, et al. Intraperitoneal lymphokine-activated killer cell/interleukin-2 therapy in patients with intra-abdominal cancer: immunologic considerations. J Nat Cancer Inst 1989; 81: 602–11.
51. Yashumoto K, Miyazaki K, Nagashima A, et al. Induction of lymphokine-activated killer cells by intrapleural instillations of recombinant interleukin-2 in patients with malignant pleurisy due to lung cancer. Cancer Res. 1987; 47: 2184–7.
52. Pizza G, Severini G, Menniti C, et al. Intralymphatic administration of interleukin-2 in cancer patients. A pilot study. Lymphokine Res 1988; 7: 45–54.
53. Abbruzzese JL, Levin B. Treatment of advanced colorectal cancer. Hem Oncol Clin N Am 1989; 3: 135–53.
54. Hamblin JJ, Davies B, Sadullah S, et al. A phase II study of the treatment of metastatic malignant melanoma with a combination of Dacarbazine, Cis-platin, Inteleukin-2 (IL2) and alfa-Interferon (IFN) in Proceed ASCO. J Clin Oncol 1991; 10: 294 (abs).
55. Demchak PA, Mier JW, Robert NJ, et al. Interleukin-2 and high dose Cisplatin in patients with metastatic melanoma: a pilot study. J Clin Oncol 1991; 9: 1821–30.
56. Rosenberg SA. The development of new immunotherapies for the treatment of cancer using Interleukin-2. Ann Surg 1988; 208: 121–35.
57. Atzpodien J, Korfer A, Franks CR, Poliwoda M, Kirchner H. Home therapy with recombinant interleukin-2 and interferon 2 in advanced malignancies. Lancet 1990; 335: 1509–12.
58. Rosenberg SA, Aebersold P, Cornetta K, et al. Gene transfer into humans: immunotherapy of patients with advanced melanoma using tumor infiltrating lymphocytes modified by retroviral gene transduction. N Engl J Med 1990; 323: 570–8.

4. Interleukin-2 toxicity: mechanisms and management

JOHANNA W. BAARS

What we know is just a drop, what we do not know an ocean.

I. Newton

Introduction

Interleukin-2 (IL-2) is a glycoprotein produced by activated T cells which is able to induce a response in 15–30% of the patients with metastatic renal cell cancer or melanoma [1–5].

This therapy is, however, accompanied by considerable side effects, including fever, chills, general malaise, nausea, vomiting, skin toxicity, hepatic and renal function disturbances, respiratory failure and haemodynamic changes resembling those observed during septic shock [1–7]. The most common side effect of (intravenously administered) IL-2 is the development of the vascular leak syndrome (VLS), which is manifested as peripheral and/or pulmonary oedema, weight gain, and occasionally ascites and/or pleural effusions [1–7]. In high dose regimens, the VLS has often been complicated by severe hypotension, oliguria and respiratory failure [1, 6, 7].

Most IL-2 toxicities appear to be dose and schedule dependent (Table 1). The highest dosing regimens often require intensive care support [1, 4, 6, 7], whereas other schemes using a lower dose of IL-2 can be managed in an oncology ward or even in the out-patient clinic [2, 3, 8, 9]. The comparison between the different dosages and schedules is made difficult by the fact that frequently the grade of the toxicities has not been well documented in the articles [1–7]. In addition, it is sometimes not clear from the text which units of IL-2 have been used. The schedule of administration also has influence on the toxicities observed during IL-2 therapy. For a certain dose of IL-2, a continuous intravenous schedule of administration is more toxic than single short infusions [10]. The local toxicities associated with other routes of administration than the intravenous route, will be described in a later section.

J. Wagstaff (ed.), The Role of Interleukin-2 in the Treatment of Cancer Patients, 45-69.

Table 1. **IL-2 toxicities. Comparison between several schedules**

Scheme	Rosenberg [1] IL-2 alone 3 dd high dose i.v.	IL-2 + LAK 3 dd high dose IL-2 i.v.	IL-2 + IFNα 3 dd high dose IL i.v.	Atzpodien [8]** IL-2 + IFNα low dose s.c. IL-2	West [2] IL-2 + LAK cont. infusion	Eberlein [3] IL-2 + LAK 3 dd low dose bolus i.v.
Number of cycles	236 cycles	348 cycles	210 cycles	52 cycles	40 patients	30 cycles
Toxicity/ fever	n.m* ± 100%	n.m.* ± 100%	n.m.* ± 100%	94%	100%	100%
Chills	32%	55%	32%	73%	100%	100%
Malaise	n.m.*	n.m.*	n.m.*	88%	100%	100%
Fatigue	n.m.*	n.m.*	n.m.*	n.m.*	100%	100%
Anorexia	n.m.*	n.m.*	n.m.*	95%	n.m.*	100%
Diarrhoea	69%	76%	56%	42%	35%	86%
Nausea/ vomiting	61%	72%	9%	50%	30%	86%
Stomatitis	2.5%+	3%	3%	n.m.*	25%	53% 7%+
Rash/ erythema	n.m.*	n.m.*	n.m.*	n.m.*	100%	54%
Pruritus	22%	23.5%	12.3%	n.m.*	n.m.*	n.m.*
Alopecia	n.m.*	n.m.*	n.m.*	13%	n.m.*	n.m.*
Hypotension requiring fluid	n.m.*	n.m.*	n.m.*	5.8%	35%	n.m.*
Requiring vasopressor support	51%	74%	19%	0%	12.5%	n.m.*
Cardiac arrhythmias	6%	11.2%	6%	3.8%	2.5%	3.3%
Myocardial infarction	1.6%	0.3%	0.5%	0%	n.m.*	0%
Angina Pectoris	2%	3%	3.8%	0%	n.m.*	0%
Respiratory distress, not intubated	7%	8%	4%	38%	16%	0%
Intubated	6%	3%	2.9%	0%	0%	3.3%[2]
Bronchospasm	0.8%	1.1%	1%	n.m.*	n.m.*	n.m.*
Pleural effusion requiring thoraco-centesis	1.7%	2.3%	0%	n.m.*	n.m.*	n.m.*
Somnolence	12%	13%	11%	0%	n.m.*	0%
Coma	4%	2.3%	4%	0%	0%	0%
Disorientation	22%	26%	24%	0%	10%	3.3%
Anaemia requiring transfusions	44%	73%	29%	0%	100%	16.6%

Table 1. Continued

Scheme	Rosenberg [1] IL-2 alone 3 dd high dose i.v.	IL-2 + LAK 3 dd high dose IL-2 i.v.	IL-2 + IFNα 3 dd high dose IL i.v.	Atzpodien [8]** IL-2 + IFNα low dose s.c. IL-2	West [2] IL-2 + LAK cont. infusion	Eberlein [3] IL-2 + LAK 3 dd low dose bolus i.v.
Number of cycles	236 cycles	348 cycles	210 cycles	52 cycles	40 patients	30 cycles
Thrombopenia						
< 20 × 10^9/l	12%	20%	1%	n.m°	n.m°	n.m.°
20–60 × 10^9	35%	43%	30%			
60–100 × 10^9/l	22%	23%	36%			
Hyperbilirubinaemia						
35–102 μmol/l	53%	55%	46%	0%[n]	12.5%	37%
103–170 μmol/l	21%	21%	5.7%			
> 171 μmol/l	11%	11.5%	2%			
Oliguria						
< 80ml/day	34%	33%	32%	0%	'Routine'	0%
80–240 ml/day	8%	3.4%	1%	0%	n.m.*	0%
Weight gain % body weight						
0–5%	45%	49%	31%	0%	32%	53%
5.1–10%	33%	43%	53%		38%	30%
10.1–15%	18%	18%	12%		30%	17%
15.1–20%	3%	4%	4%		12%	0%
> 20.1%	1%	2%	0%		0%	0%
Creat in μmol/l						
187–534 μmol/l	63%	68%	58%	n.m.*	> 267 μmol/l	46.6%
535–890 μmol/l	9%	10%	7%		30%	
> 891 μmol/l	2%	0.6%	0.5%			
Thyroid dysfunction	n.m.*	n.m.*	n.m.*	37%	n.m.*	n.m.*
Central line sepsis	5.5%	10.3%	3.3%	–	2.5%	6.6%
Mortality	1.7%	0.9%	0.5%	0%	2.5%	0%

* N.m. = not exactly mentioned
** Only Atzpodien et al. mentioned the WHO grade of the toxicities
\+ Severe mucositis, requiring liquid diet
° N.m. = not exactly mentioned, no platelet-transfusion required
² Vocal cord oedema, requiring tracheostoma
ⁿ Forty one % elevations of transaminases and other liver enzymes not exceeding WHO grade III

The mechanisms by which IL-2 induces its side effects are largely unknown. Studies in animal models have demonstrated the central role of an intact immune system in mediating many of the toxicities [11]. The adverse effects of IL-2 are thought to be mediated by other cytokines whose production is stimulated by IL-2 [12–17], by the direct toxic effects of stimulated lymphocytes on the endothelium [7] and by the secondary induction of other mediator systems, such as the complement system [18] and production of phospholipase A2 [19] (Figure 1).

Considerable effort has been put into the elucidation of the exact nature of IL-2 toxicity. These data will be discussed in detail in relation to the specific toxicities observed during IL-2 treatment. This will be followed by several management-guidelines and possible means of ameliorating the adverse effects of IL-2.

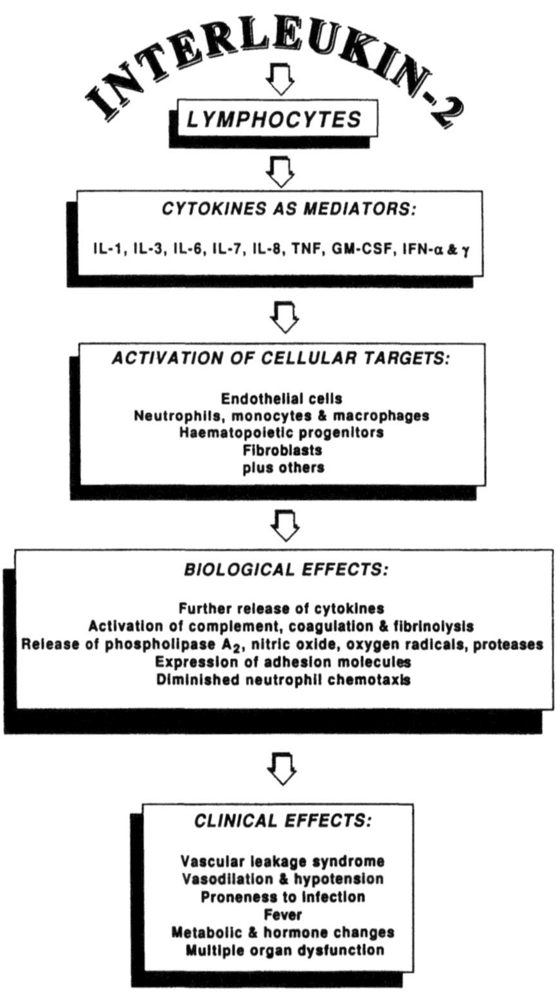

Figure 1. Highly simplified scheme, showing some of the mechanisms by which IL-2 can induce its side effects.

IL-2 Induced toxicities and hypotheses about their pathogenesis

The vascular leak syndrome (VLS)

One of the major complications of IL-2 treatment is an increased vascular permeability causing a leakage of fluid from the intravascular into the interstitial space of many organs [1–7].

Fluid accumulation in the lung is an especially troublesome toxicity leading to considerable morbidity for the patients [1–7], causing respiratory insufficiency requiring oxygen supplementation and occasionally ventilatory support [1–7]. A similar increase in vascular leakage has been observed in mice [11, 20]. In the murine system, a clear relationship between the degree of VLS and the dose and duration of IL-2 administration has been demonstrated [11, 20]. The same holds true for humans [1–7]. In mice, the VLS was most pronounced in the thymus, spleen, lungs, liver and kidneys [11].

The mechanisms by which IL-2 can exert its influences on vascular permeability are complicated and despite extensive research are not completely understood. A direct toxic effect of IL-2 on the blood vessels is not likely, since nude and irradiated mice treated with IL-2 did not show any vascular leakage [11, 20].

There is one study suggesting that IL-2 can exert a direct toxic effect on blood vessels in the lungs of rats, but the lungs were removed before IL-2 infusion and the results obtained are therefore difficult to interpret [21]. It seems more likely that IL-2 induces the VLS indirectly through activation of other pathways, including generation or induction of vasoactive substances, release of other cytokines and the generation of activated cells causing toxicity to the blood vessels.

Studies in mice have shown that lymphokine activated killer (LAK) cells and their continued stimulation by IL-2 in vivo may play a role in the mediation of VLS [20, 22]. Selective depletion of various lymphoid subsets using monoclonal antibodies has been used to identify the cell population involved in production of the VLS [20, 22]. It became apparent that natural killer (NK) cells/LAK precursors, but not transferred activated T cells were required for the development of VLS [20, 22]. The mechanism by which these cells cause or contribute to the damage of vascular tissues remains to be elucidated. LAK cells may directly adhere to endothelial cells and subsequently lyse them or they may produce other factors that may damage the endothelium.

Exposure of lymphocytes to IL-2 in vitro rapidly induces their ability to adhere to human endothelial cells, causing endothelial injury [23]. The ability of IL-2 to induce NK cell adhesion to endothelial cells was not blocked by a mixture of neutralising antisera raised against recombinant (r) tumour necrosis factor alpha (TNF-α), r Interleukin-1 alpha or beta (rIL-1α, rIL-1β), factors which are known to promote leukocyte adhesion to endothelial cells [23]. In one study LAK cells from human peripheral blood, but not LAK culture supernatant or IL-1, IL-2, IL-3, IL-4, IL-6, TNF, Granulocyte-Monocyte

Colony Stimulating Factor (GM-CSF), Interferon-gamma (IFN-γ) increased the permeability of an endothelial cell monolayer for fluorescein labeled albumin [24]. This study suggests the direct involvement of LAK cells in mediating increased vascular permeability. The ability of LAK cells to lyse endothelial cells after in vitro culture may not, however, reflect their ability to lyse endothelial cells in vivo. Ferro et al. [25] showed that the increased vascular permeability in pulmonary vessels occurred indepently of circulating lymphocytes and was related to thromboxane A2 (T× A2) generation upon IL-2 administration. LAK cells in vivo did not show significant endothelial cytolysis at effector to target ratios of 100:1 in an ovine model [26]. The increased endothelial monolayer permeability to albumin was, however, dependent on the concentration of LAK cells. These findings suggest that the VLS is mediated by LAK cells in vivo via non-cytolytic mechanisms and/or the release of secondary cytokines in response to IL-2 [26]. Cotran et al. [27] have shown that administration of IL-2 leads to wide-spread endothelial activation as evidenced by enhanced expression of endothelial-leucocyte adhesion molecule 1, intercellular adhesion molecule 1 and HLA-DQ. The expression of these molecules is associated with increased vascular permeability [27]. Although IL-2 cannot induce expression of activation antigens on endothelial cells in vitro, cytokines induced by IL-2, for example TNF-α and IFN-γ [12–15], are able to induce this phenomenon [27]. TNF-α and IFN-γ have been shown to induce morphologic and behavioral changes in endothelial cells in vitro, which may underlie vascular lesions in vivo [28]. TNF might also contribute to the VLS by stimulating production of other agents, like phospholipase-A2, which increases vascular permeability. The effects of TNF-α on the induction of VLS are, however, not entirely clear and elucidated, because both in vitro and in vivo studies fail to show any enhancement of vascular permeability due to TNF [24, 29, 30]. Interferon-alpha (IFN-α), IFN-γ, TNF-α and IL-1 were not able to induce vascular leakage in the lungs of mice, when administered alone [29, 31]. The combination of IL-2 and IFN-α induced more severe VLS in mice than IL-2 alone [29], while IL-1α decreased the VLS [31]. The mechanisms of these phenomena are not clear. IFN-α can lead to enhanced LAK activity and IL-1α increases endothelial proliferation which might make the endothelium less susceptible to IL-2 toxicity [7].

Other mediator systems might also play a contributory role in the development of the VLS. As in septic shock, the complement system becomes activated during IL-2 treatment [18], which can cause endothelial damage. The concentration of the activated third component of the complement system appeared to be correlated with the degree of weight-gain, decrease in albumin and hypotension [18, 32]. There also existed a clear relationship between the dose of IL-2 administered to the patient and the plasma concentration of the activated third component of the complement system [18].

During IL-2 treatment, the complement system is activated both by the alternative and classical pathways [33]. The hepatic acute phase reactant C-reactive protein, which is shown to be released during IL-2 treatment, is thought to play a contributory role in the induction of complement activation via the classical route [33].

In rats, a constant infusion but not a rapid bolus administration of IL-2 produces multiple-system oedema, increased thromboxane B2 plasma-levels, sequestration of polymorphonuclear neutrophils (PMN) in the lungs and enhanced microvascular permeability [34]. It is well known that activated PMN contribute to the clinical signs and symptoms of the septic shock syndrome [35], which resembles IL-2 toxicity. Indeed, PMN also become activated during IL-2 treatment, as evidenced by enhanced neutrophil elastase and lactoferrin plasma levels [32]. PMN can secrete toxic oxygen radicals and other proteases, which might cause endothelial damage. There existed, however, no relationship between the elastase and lactoferrin levels and parameters of the VLS [32]. Other agents, known to increase vascular permeability such as histamine or serotonine do not appear to play a major role in the induction of VLS, since antagonists fail to ameliorate this syndrome [7].

In summary, the VLS is one of the major complications of IL-2 therapy. The mechanisms by which IL-2 induces vascular leakage are not clear. LAK cells, the release of other cytokines, activation of other mediators systems such as the complement system, activation of PMN, release of agents which enhance vascular permeability, for example phospholipase A2, might all play a contributory role.

Cardiovascular toxicity

A variety of cardiac side effects have been observed during IL-2 treatment, especially with high dose regimens [1, 6, 7, 36, 37]. These toxicities include tachycardia, arrhythmias, ischaemia, myocarditis, hypocontractibility and pericardial effusions [1, 6, 7, 36–38]. IL-2 administration causes reversible haemodynamic changes and left ventricular dysfunction similar to those seen in septic shock. Decreased mean arterial blood pressure, increased cardiac index and decreased peripheral vascular resistance are all present during intensive IL-2 treatment [37, 39]. In addition, the left ventricular ejection fraction decreases which is associated with a trend toward left ventricular dilatation as manifested by an increase in left ventricular and diastolic volume index [37, 39]. Although the blood pressure normalised within 24 hours of discontinuation of IL-2 therapy, the systemic vascular resistance remained below baseline levels for 6 days after IL-2 treatment had been discontinued [39].

Supraventricular tachycardias including atrial fibrillation are the most common arrhythmias observed during intensive IL-2 regimens and occur in 10% or more of patients [1, 4–7, 35]. These toxicities generally resolve after discontinuation of IL-2.

Dangerous ventricular arrhythmias and sudden death have also been observed, especially in patients experiencing myocardial ischaemia [1, 6, 7, 39]. Myocardial ischaemia occurred in 3% to 9% and myocardial infarction in 1% to 4% of the patients treated with high dose IL-2 regimens [1, 7, 36, 40]. The frequency of these complications is influenced by patient selection and the used treatment schedule. Careful screening of the patients to rule out underlying coronary disease might reduce the incidence of myocardial complications during (high dose) IL-2 therapy [7].

ECG changes and CPK-MB elevations with or without chest pain have also been observed in young individuals without evidence of coronary disease [41], and may therefore be due to IL-2 induced coronary artery spasm, non-ischaemic myocardial injury or myocarditis.

There is no evidence that IL-2 exerts a direct effect on the myocardium. In vitro studies with isolated rat hearts have shown that neither IL-2 alone nor mononuclear cells directly induced cardiotoxicity [42, 43]. The study of Sobotka et al. [42] suggested that IL-2 stimulated human mononuclear cells produce soluble factor(s) which induces reversible severe depression of cardiac function. The proteins made by activated mononuclear cells are numerous and can include TNF-α and IL-1. These cytokines have been shown to influence the contractility of cultured myocytes [44].

In a rabbit model, IL-2 treatment resulted in perivascular and interstitial infiltration of the myocardium by lymphocytes but no attendant necrosis [16]. Lymphocytic infiltration can play a role in IL-2 induced cardiac toxicity, but it remains to be proven whether this is the case in the human situation.

Hypotension requiring administration of fluids and/or vasopressor support is a common toxicity in patients receiving IL-2 therapy and is often dose limiting [1–7, 36, 37, 39]. It can result from depressed cardiac contractility, decrease of peripheral vascular resistance and decreased intravascular volume due to the VLS.

The pathogenesis of IL-2 induced hypotension is complex and not entirely elucidated. Because the haemodynamic changes observed during IL-2 treatment resemble those seen during the septic shock syndrome, it is likely that mediator systems activated in septicaemia might also play a role in IL-2 induced toxicities. Considerable evidence has been accumulated to indicate that increased vascular permeability in combination with vasodilatation are central events in the development of septic shock [45, 46]. As with IL-2 treatment, endothelial cell activation and/or damage are thought to be mediated via in vivo generation of cytokines such as IL-1, TNF-α, IFN-γ [45, 46]. Vasodilatation has been attributed to activation of the complement cascade and the contact (intrinsic coagulation) system with subsequent release of anaphylatoxins such as C3a, C5a and bradykinin [35, 46, 47]. As already mentioned, the complement system is activated during IL-2 treatment [18, 33] and there existed a clear correlation between the degree of hypotension and the plasma concentration of C3a [18].

The contact system is also activated during intensive IL-2 treatment [48]. The role of this system in IL-2 induced hypotension has to be further clarified.

In sepsis and during IL-2 treatment the endothelial and myocardial damage might be in part mediated by the release of proteases and the generation of toxic oxygen species by marginated PMN, that are activated by endogenous cytokines and products of the complement cascade [35, 46, 49].

Recent studies suggest that nitric oxide produced by macrophages and endothelial cells might play a role in the induction of hypotension during septicaemia and treatment with cytokines [46, 50–52]. Indeed, an IFN-γ, TNF and IL-1 inducible pathway synthesising nitric oxide from arginine has been demonstrated in patients receiving high dose IL-2 [53]. An inhibitor of nitric oxide synthesis, N^G-methyl-L-arginine could reverse the endotoxin-mediated hypotension in dogs [52], suggesting that nitric oxide overproduction might be an important contributor to the septic shock syndrome and might be also responsible for some of the toxicities observed during IL-2 treatment. Inhibitors of nitric oxide synthesis might be of therapeutic value in the treatment of cytokine induced hypotension, provided this has no negative influence on anti-tumour efficacy.

Pulmonary toxicity

The VLS contributes much to the pulmonary toxicities observed during IL-2 treatment, causing lung oedema and occasionally pleural effusions,requiring thoracocentesis [1, 4, 6, 7, 36, 39]. In studies with high dose regimens, approximately 20% of the patients developed respiratory distress and 5–10% required intubation and mechanical ventilation [1, 6, 7]. Most patients have lung oedema with normal or even low left atrial pressure, indicating that this phenomenon is likely to be caused by increased vascular permeability rather than fluid overload due to a poor cardiac function or inadvertent intravenous fluid administration [1, 6, 7, 36, 39]. This toxicity is reversible upon discontinuation of treatment in the majority of patients. Reversible bronchospasm has also been observed in patients undergoing IL-2 therapy.

Animal studies have shown that the lung vasculature is very sensitive to IL-2 induced toxicity, since the increase in vascular permeability was greater in the lungs than in many other organs [11, 54].

Sheep, infused with IL-2, showed a dose-dependent significant decrease in arterial pO_2, an increase in high-protein lymph flow and infiltration of lymphoblastoid cells into the lung parenchyma [55]. Accumulation of macrophages and lymphocytes in the alveolar septae together with increased vascular leakage have been also observed in mice [11, 56].

The study of Klausner et al. [57] indicated that IL-2 induced pulmonary hypertension was mediated by thromboxane A2, partly derived from neutrophils. It is possible that lymphocytic infiltration and thromboxane A2 also contribute to IL-2 induced pulmonary toxicity in humans.

Nephrotoxicity

Renal dysfunction is a common complication of IL-2 therapy [1–7], characterised by azotemia, oliguria, very low sodium excretion and elevated plasma renin activity [58–60]. Prerenal mechanisms are thought to be the cause of these abnormalities in renal function, the renal perfusion being impaired due to reduced cardiac function, peripheral vascular dilatation and intravascular volume depletion due to the VLS [7]. The results of the radionuclide studies performed by Shalmi et al. [61] suggest that, in addition to a major prerenal component, an intrinsic intrarenal defect might also contribute to the renal dysfunction, as evidenced by an absence of a marked increase in the ureum/creatinine ratio [61]. Most nephrotoxicity resolves after therapy is completed, although occasionally recovery may be prolonged and/or incomplete [59, 62]. Impaired renal function before therapy increases the likelihood of severe and prolonged nephrotoxicity [61]. Acute tubular necrosis is seldom observed during IL-2 treatment [53]. Cytokine induced nitric oxide production in the renal parenchyma might protect the kidney against this complication by maintaining postglomerular circulation [53]. Administration of non-steroidal anti-inflammatory drugs (NSAID's) can contribute to the impairment of renal function [63]. Nephrotoxic drugs should be avoided in patients receiving IL-2.

Gastro-intestinal and hepatic toxicity

Gastro-intestinal toxicities due to IL-2 therapy include nausea, vomiting and/or diarrhoea [1–7, 64]. Stomatitis is a common problem, sometimes requiring a liquid diet [1–7]. Occasionally localised necrosis or perforation of the colon during high dose IL-2 treatment has been observed [64]. Although the causes of the colonic perforations and infarctions are unknown, impaired perfusion due to hypotension, tissue oedema and vasoconstriction due to pressor agents are likely to be contributory factors.

During high dose IL-2 treatment acute pancreatitis has been described, but this complication is rare [65]. Stress-induced gastric acid secretion and the administration of NSAID's to control fever predispose patients receiving IL-2 to the development of peptic ulcer disease [6].

Intra-hepatic cholestasis with elevation of bilirubin is observed in patients receiving IL-2 [1–7, 66]. Elevations of other liver enzymes and prolonged prothrombin time are also common [1–7, 66]. The pathophysiologic mechanisms of these hepatic function disturbances are unknown. The cholestasis observed in patients receiving high-dose IL-2 is intrahepatic and likely to be related to disturbed canalicular bile flow [66].

Hepatocytes are not known to express IL-2 receptors, but numerous lymphoid cells which may express such receptors exist within the liver and could mediate some of the toxicity [66]. Tissue bound macrophages can contribute to the hepatotoxicity because they can be stimulated by cytokines released during IL-2 treatment, such as IFN-γ [14]. Also other cytokines released during IL-2 treatment, such as TNF [12, 13, 15] and IL-6 [67] might mediate some of the liver function changes.

Endocrinologic and metabolic toxicity

The neuroendocrine system and the immune system are closely connected with each other and cytokines play an important role in the complex interplay between these systems [68]. It is therefore not surprising that treatment with IL-2 causes alterations in the neuroendocrine system.

Thyroid dysfunction has been described in patients treated with IL-2, ranging from hypothyroidism to hyperthyroïdism, sometimes associated with a goiter [7, 8, 69, 70]. The frequency of this complication depends on the mode of IL-2 administration and combination with other cytokines such as IFN-α, which by itself can also induce thyroid dysfunction [71, 72]. Many patients had or developed antimicrosomal antibodies. In one study, thyroid toxicity seemed to be correlated with tumour response [69]. The thyroid dysfunction is thought to be based on induction of auto-immune processes by IL-2 treatment. It has been postulated that IFN-γ plays an important role in both sporadic and cytokine induced thyroid dysfunction through its ability to induce the expression of HLA Class II antigens [73] and adhesion molecules on thyrocytes [74], which allows these cells to present their thyroid antigens effectively to T lymphocytes. Paradoxically, longterm IFN-γ treatment did not result in the development of thyroid abnormalities [75]. Moreover, IFN-γ protected in vitro human thyroid epithelial cells against cell mediated cytotoxicity [76]. Another hypothesis can be proposed based on the recently reported thyroid dysfunction during treatment with granulocyte-monocyte-colony stimulating factor (GM-CSF) production [77]. GM-CSF can prime antigen-presenting cells to a state in which they can activate auto-aggressive T cell clones, leading ultimately to the induction of thyroid autoimmunity [77]. Treatment with IL-2 induces GM-CSF production [77, 78], which might contribute to thyroid dysfunctions. Direct actions of cytokines on the hypothalamic-pituitary-thyroid axis have been described. IL-1, TNF, IFN-γ and IFN-α can inhibit this axis, acting at different levels [68]. The results of in vitro experiments are, however, controversial, depending on the dose of the cytokine used and the experimental conditions [68]. The IL-2 induced thyroid dysfunction is in most cases self limiting after discontinuation of IL-2 treatment [69].

Corticotropin, cortisol, prolactin, growth hormone and beta-endorphin levels have been shown to be elevated after administration of IL-2 [79–81]. The elevation of cortisol levels may be of particular significance, since steroid hormones have the potential of modulating the response to IL-2 [82]. The release of these hormones is likely to be induced by activation of the hypothalamic-pituitary axis by IL-1, IL-6, TNF and IL-2 itself [68]. In vitro experiments have shown that IL-1, IL-2 and IL-6 can directly influence the function of adrenal cells, but the results are unequivocal [68]. It has been reported that elevations of beta endorphin, corticotropin and cortisol are of far greater magnitude after re-exposure to IL-2 following a 6 day to 3 month interval than after the initial cycle [81]. The mechanisms of this anamnestic response is unknown. The finding that at least some physiologic responses remain altered as a result of IL-2 therapy received weeks or months earlier might have important therapeutic implications.

Adrenal haemorrhage with acute adrenal insufficiency has occurred in a patient with renal adenocarcinoma and bilateral adrenal involvement with tumour while receiving IL-2 therapy [83]. The exact cause of this event is not known. Close clinical observation appears to be prudent in the management of patients with adrenal metastases during IL-2 based therapies, since these patients are prone to develop this toxicity. It is a dangerous complication, because many signs and symptoms of adrenal insufficiency resemble the side effects of IL-2, while lack of endogenous steroid production may render patients at risk for severe IL-2 toxicity.

During treatment with high dose IL-2 a reversible acute hypocholesterolaemia has been observed with virtual disappearance of high-density lipoproteins and a marked reduction in the concentration of low density lipoproteins (LDL) [84]. The remaining LDL and intermediate-density lipoproteins were enriched in triglyceride relative to cholesterol and had broad β electrophoretic modality. These changes differed from those reported for other cytokines such as TNF or the IFN's [84]. The pathogenesis of this toxicity is not clear. Secondary release of other cytokines, changes in hormone secretion and hepatotoxicity might all play a role.

Mucocutaneous toxicities

Cutaneous toxicities due to IL-2 include macular erythema, pruritus, generalised erythrodermia and desquamation, the latter particularly of the distal extremities [1–7, 85].

Pruritus and desquamation can last for several weeks after discontinuation of the treatment. The histological changes are non-specific, consisting of lymphoid cells surrounding blood vessels in the papillary dermis with fewer of these cells in the epidermis, focal vacuolar basal cell degeneration and rare scattered necrotic keratinocytes [85]. The lymphoid cells were mostly of the CD4+/HLA-DR+ phenotype. Sporadic cases of IL-2 associated erythema nodosum, fatal pemphigus vulgaris and life threatening bullous skin lesions have been reported [86–89]. The patient who experienced fatal pemphigus vulgaris was also treated with IFN-β and the patients with life threatening bullous skin lesions were receiving antibiotics. Whether these agents have contributed to the skin toxicity is not clear.

Exacerbations of psoriasis [90] and of polymyositis/ dermatomyositis [7] have been reported in patients with pre-existing disease. As with the endocrinologic toxicities, several of these dermatological phenomena are likely to reflect autoimmune processes induced or augmented by IL-2 or might be induced by direct effects of cytokines on the skin. During IL-2 treatment, especially with the continuous mode of administration, we have occasionally observed a slight conjuctivitis rapidly resolving upon discontinuation of treatment.

Neurologic toxicities

Disturbances in concentration, sleepiness and disorientation are common during IL-2 therapy [1–7, 91]. Other reported toxicities are agitation, somnolence, coma, hallucinations and seizures [1, 6, 7, 91], especially during high dose IL-2 therapy. It has been observed that such mental status changes often progress even in the first days after discontinuation of therapy [1, 6, 7, 91].

It has been proposed that these neurologic function disturbances might be due to increased cerebral water content, secondary cytokine release or damage to the blood-brain barrier [7]. IL-2 infusion in cats caused, within the perivascular brain parenchyma, numerous disrupted neuronal and glial processes as well as expanded intercellular spaces [92]. Since animals which received only the excipient of IL-2 also showed changes in the morphology of the blood-brain barrier, it is difficult to distinguish which changes were caused by the IL-2 and which changes were due to the excipient or study methods.

Hyperaesthesias and paraesthesias have also been noted in patients on IL-2 therapy [7]. Furthermore, transient ischaemic attacks and cerebrovascular accidents have occurred during IL-2 administration [7].

Because the signs and symptoms of cerebral metastases or cerebral tumours can deteriorate during systemic IL-2 treatment due to oedema in the metastases or tumour consequent to the VLS, it might be wise to exclude these patients from IL-2 based studies [93].

Spinal cord compression due to enlargement of metastatic sites caused by oedema has been described [94]. The patients should be screened for metastatic sites where sudden enlargement would compromise physiological function.

Haematologic toxicity and coagulation disturbances

Haematologic changes observed during IL-2 therapy include anaemia, transient lymphopenia followed by rebound lymphocytosis after discontinuation of treatment, eosinophilia, thrombocytopenia and occasional transient granulocytopenia [1–7, 95]. Lymphopenia is most commonly observed early in intensive therapy and is probably attributable to margination [1, 6, 7, 95]. The alteration in lymphocyte number may be mediated directly by IL-2. IL-2 produced a significant decline in circulating erythroid and granulocytic-macrophage progenitors, which rebounded after cessation of IL-2 therapy [95]. This IL-2 mediated suppression of haematopoiesis might be due to secondary release of other cytokines, for example the interferons [95]. The hematopoiesis during IL-2 treatment is, however, not only influenced by cytokines which have an inhibitory effect on this process, but is also regulated by the release of interleukin-5 (IL-5), GM-CSF, monocyte colony-stimulating factor (M-CSF), granulocyte colony-stimulating factor (G-CSF) and IL-6 [78, 96, 97]. The induction of IL-5, G-CSF, GM-CSF during IL-2 treatment can account for the neutrophilia and eosinophilia observed in patients undergoing IL-2 therapy. IL-

2 based regimens can also induce auto-antibody formation against erythrocytes and thrombocytes [98], leading to haemolytic anaemia or thrombocytopenia.

The administration of IL-2 causes the release of TNF [12, 13, 15) which, by disturbing the anticoagulant properties of the endothelium [99, 100], may induce a procoagulant state in patients receiving this drug. IL-2 activates the coagulation and fibrinolytic systems in a way resembling the pertubations observed after endotoxin and TNF administration [99, 101, 133]. The procoagulant state induced by IL-2 might contribute to organ dysfunction or by disturbing blood flow in tumour vasculature, might exert influence on anti-tumour efficacy. Apart from the induction of changes in the coagulation state at the endothelial cell level, high dose IL-2 treatment also interferes with hepatic synthesis of clotting factors and their inhibitors [102].

Fever, chills and constitutional symptoms

Fever and chills occur in almost every patient who receives IL-2 irrespective of the dose and schedule used [1–7]. It is thought that IL-2 for itself is not a pyrogen but probably causes fever by inducing release of other cytokines like TNF, IL-1 and IL-6 [7, 12–15]. Many patients experience flu-like symptoms such as headache, myalgia, arthralgia, general malaise and fatigue [1–7]. These phenomena are rarely severe and can be treated symptomatically.

Exacerbation of antoimmune diseases

IL-2 and other cytokines may be important in the pathogenesis of antibody and cell mediated auto-immune disease. Increased levels of IL-2 have recently been found in the sera of patients with sclerodermia, showing some correlation with disease activity [103]. Elevated levels of IFN-γ, correlating with disease activity, have been found in the sera of patients with systemic lupus erythematosus [104].

Autoimmune toxicites induced by IL-2 have been mentioned in the former sections. It is likely that IL-2 administration to patients with active autoimmune disorders might lead to exacerbation of their disease.

Infections

The incidence of bacterial infections during IL-2 therapy varies between 0 to 40% [7, 105, 106]. Infectious complications do not only occur in patients receiving high dose IL-2 regimens, but have also been described in patients undergoing subcutaneous treatment in an outpatient setting [105]. The organisms most frequently involved are Staphylococcus aureus and epidermidis [7, 105, 106], although gram negative infections can also occur during IL-2 treatment [105, 107]. Patients may have positive blood cultures in absence of an overt infection [107]. This might be dangerous, because the symptoms and signs of infections are often masked by IL-2 induced toxicity. Apart from predisposing factors such as the presence of a central venous catheter, intravesical devices, administration of in vitro cultured lymphocytes and the dermatologic toxicity of IL-2, several lines of evidence suggest that IL-2 treatment temporarily alters the immune-response causing an increased susceptibility to infections, especially with staphylococci [7, 106, 108]. Transient impairment of cell mediated immunity as measured by response to recall antigens as well as a decrease in in vitro lymphocyte proliferation after IL-2 have been reported [109]. The neutrophil function is influenced by IL-2 therapy as evidenced by diminished respiratory burst in response to classic stimuli, decreased Fc receptor expression [110] and a decreased neutrophil chemotaxis [111]. It has also been suggested that IL-2 may impair phagocytic cell function [109]. The mechanisms of the induction of these defects are not known. TNF which, as already noted, is released during IL-2 treatment can cause similar neutrophil dysfunction in vitro [7].

Promotion of tumour growth

It is not clear whether IL-2 exacerbates growth and progression of some malignancies, either by acting as a growth factor or through immunomodulation. It is known that leukaemic cell lines have IL-2 receptors and some of these will proliferate in vitro in response to IL-2 [7, 112]. Furthermore, it is possible that IL-2 can promote tumour growth indirectly by induction of release of other cytokines such as TNF, IL-1, IL-6 and IFN-γ, which can have in vitro tumour growth promoting effects [112].

Toxicities related to the mode of administration

Apart from the intravenous mode of administration, IL-2 may be given intra-arterially, subcutaneously, intraperitoneally, intrapleurally and directly into tumour tissue.

Substantial systemic toxicities have been observed during intra-arterial IL-2 administration at doses higher than 18×10^6 International Units/m^2/day as continuous infusion [113]. In addition, both vascular variations and catheter-related problems consisting frequently of thrombosis of the artery, compromise this treatment approach [114].

During intraperitoneal administration of IL-2 abdominal pain, colonic perforation and a grand mal seizure have been observed, apart from systemic toxicities [115]. Fourteen out of twenty four patients developed intraperitoneal fibrosis. It was noted that during this treatment the numbers of eosinophils increased in the peritoneal cavity [115]. Eosinophils can secrete eosinophil major basic protein, a substance which stimulates collagen synthesis. In addition, IL-1 and Tumour Growth Factor-β (TGFβ) can contribute to the development of fibrosis, also by stimulating collagen synthesis [115].

Intrapleural administration of IL-2 was usually well tolerated [116, 117].

Intratumoural IL-2 administered to patients with gliomas can result in the development of cerebral oedema around the site of treatment, grade III-IV

WHO fever, increased cerebral pressure, confusion and aseptic meningitis [118, 119]. Subcutaneous injections of IL-2 can cause redness, swelling and pain at the place of administration, which was reported to be tolerated by the patients [8]. During local treatment of the bladder with IL-2, no significant toxicity has been observed [120].

Mortality due to IL-2 treatment

The mortality rate due to high dose IL-2 treatment is reported to be between 1–3% [1, 6, 7]. The causes of death were septicaemia, myocardial infarction and lung embolism [1, 4–7].

Development of antibodies to IL-2

Long-term use of genetically engineered proteins in humans can result in specific antibody formation. Although neutralising antibodies to recombinant IL-2 have been reported in a few patients receiving long-term IL-2 [121], the biological and clinical effects of antibody formation are yet to be defined.

Most patients treated with recombinant IL-2 receive short-term therapy. Therefore IL-2 antibody formation may not be as important as the antigenicity of other recombinant proteins which are used chronically (e.g. insulin, IFN-α). Because of the severe toxicity from high-dose IL-2, other schemes have, however, been developed using low-dose longterm IL-2. Recent studies have shown that combined subcutaneous application of recombinant IL-2 and IFN-α led to significant enhancement of the production of anti IL-2 antibodies [8, 122]. The development of neutralising antibodies might lead to a significant decrease in biological activation [121], which may have consequences for the anti-tumour efficacy of this therapy. This can be overcome by using higher doses of recombinant IL-2 in vitro or administration of natural IL-2 in vivo. Antibody formation against natural IL-2 has been seldom observed [122] and the clinical consequences of this phenomenon have to be defined.

Amelioration of IL-2 toxicity

It is not exactly known by which mechanisms IL-2 causes anti-tumour efficacy and toxicity. Therefore, the question whether endeavours to reduce IL-2 toxicity will also cause a decrease in anti-tumour efficacy remains to be answered. Careful selection of patients participating in IL-2 trials and good supportive care can contribute to the prevention and/or reduction of the IL-2 induced side effects.

There is a clear relationship between the dose and schedule of IL-2 used and the observed toxicities. The high dose IL-2 regimens developed by Rosenberg et al. [1] are based on the observation in animal models that the anti-tumour efficacy correlated closely with the dose of IL-2 used and the number of infused LAK-cells [123, 124]. Also the duration of IL-2 therapy might be of importance for induction of antitumour response [10]. West et al. [2] obtained a similar response rate with a continuous infusion of IL-2, using approximately 25% of the dose of IL-2 administered by Rosenberg et al. [1], but the scheme still causes considerable toxicity [2]. Indeed, a recent randomised study comparing the anti-tumour efficacy and toxicity of the Rosenberg and West scheme showed nearly similar side effects and serious complications [125].

Atzpodien et al. [8] developed a subcutaneous treatment schedule which can be managed at the out-patient clinic with tolerable and moderate side effects in a selective patient population with a good performance status and often small tumour loads. In our experience, the toxicity of the subcutaneous schedule is of a greater magnitude than Atzpodien described, the patients experiencing a moderate to severe reduction in general well being. The merits of this scheme must be further explored, also in respect to its anti-tumour response.

Pretreatment with cyclophosphamide, a cytoreductive agent with immunomodulating properties, has been shown to decrease IL-2 toxicity in mice [7, 11, 20, 126, 127]. The results of this pretreatment in humans are equivocal [9, 128]. Mitchell et al. [9] observed no toxicity above WHO grade III and could manage the scheme in the out-patient clinic whereas Lindemann et al. [128], who administered the IL-2 for a longer period, could not detect protection by cyclophosphamide pretreatment from IL-2 induced toxicity, with the vascular leak syndrome, myalgia and fever being the greatest problems.

Corticosteroids eliminate much of the toxicity attributable to IL-2 therapy but may also decrease its efficacy [82]. As already mentioned, TNF is thought to be an important mediator of IL-2 toxicity. Mier et al. [129] have shown that concurrent administration of dexamethasone with IL-2 prevented the in vivo generation of TNF, resulting in amelioration of the vascular leak syndrome and the degree of hypotension observed after IL-2 infusion. In addition, passive immunisation against TNF can partially abrogate IL-2 toxicity in animals [130]. Neutralising antibodies to cytokines which are released during IL-2 may improve tolerance to this therapy. It is, however, not known to what extent the action of such cytokines is required to achieve the desired therapeutic responses to IL-2. For example, Blay et al. [131] have shown that there was a correlation between clinical response to IL-2 therapy and sustained release of TNF upon discontinuation of treatment in patients with metastatic renal cell cancer.

On the other hand, concomitant IL-2 administration with other cytokines, especially IL-1 and TNF-α may protect against IL-2 induced VLS [30, 31]. IL-1α has been shown to have such an effect in a mouse model [31]. The study of Mier et al. [30] suggested that TNF-α and IL-1 increased endothelial resistance in vitro to LAK cell lysis. In a recent preliminary report, it was indicated that sequential administration of TNF-α and IL-2 to cancer patients resulted in less toxicity than did administration of IL-2 alone [132]. Concomitant IL-2 administration with other cytokines might also enhance toxicity. As already mentioned, combined treatment of IFN-α and IL-2 resulted in the enhancement of the VLS and related toxicities in mice in comparison to IL-2 alone [29].

Further studies are needed to determine what is the optimal timing of such combination therapy, whether treatment with IL-1 and/or TNF-α protects patients from serious toxicities of IL-2 and what effect these combinations have on the efficacy of therapy. Because an activated complement system and activated neutrophils might contribute to IL-2 toxicity, especially the VLS and hypotension [18, 32], it might be worthwhile to try to ameliorate the side effects with complement 1-esterase inhibitor or superoxide-dismutase, although the effects of such an intervention on anti-tumour response have to be defined.

The same holds true for the administration of inhibitors of nitric oxide synthesis in hope of ameliorating IL-2 induced hypotension, although this might also have adverse consequences for the renal function [53].The symptomatic treatment of IL-2 induced toxicity is summarised in Table 2.

Table 2. Symptomatic management of IL-2 induced toxicity

Toxicity	Management
Hypotension	– Administration of fluids: limit daily positive fluid balance to < 1.5 liters – Vasopressors: low dopamine 3–5 μg/kg/ min to maintain urine output, start phenylepinephrine early 1–5 μg/kg/min for hypotension not responsive to 15 μg/kg/min dopamine
Weight gain/oedema	– Limit fluids, furosemide as tolerated by blood pressure
Cardiac toxicities	
Arrhythmias	– SVT: medical therapy, continue IL-2 – Unsustained VT or frequent PVC's: medical therapy, continue IL-2 – Sustained VT or any arrhythmia requiring cardioversion: discontinue IL-2
Cardiac ischaemia	– Discontinue IL-2, rule out myocardial infarction – N.B.: any severe onset of hypotension or pulmonary oedema may be cardiogenic rather than simply attributable to IL-2
Pulmonary toxicity	– Limit fluids – Oxygen, bronchodilatators if indicated – Diuretics if tolerated by bloodpressure – Early intubation in the presence of deterioration
Neurotoxicity	– Agitation: benzodiazepines, antihistamines, psychological support – Correct contributing metabolic factors – Confusion, psychosis, severe agitation: discontinue IL-2 treatment – Watch for late onset or progression after cessation of IL-2
Infection	– Culture blood and any suspicious sites – Severe acidosis may be a sign of sepsis; other IL-2 toxcities may be exacerbated by sepsis – Empiric coverage must be directed at staphylococci species – Prophylactic antibodies if central venous line is necessary

Table 2. Continued

Toxicity	Management
Gastrointestinal side effects	
Nausea/vomiting	- Antiemetics, e.g. metoclopramide, 5HT3 antagonists
Diarrhoea	- Loperamide, diet
Stomatitis	- Symptomatically, liquid diet - Total parenteral nutritions if necessary - Watch for bowel perforation
Fever, chills, constitutional symptoms	- Acetaminophen - NSAID's: watch for deterioration of renal function - Morphine analogues for severe chills
Pruritus	- Antihistamines - Symptomatic treatment - Unguentum leniens in case of dry skin with desquamation
Thyroid	- Depending on clinical signs and symptoms; temporary thyroxine suppletion is sometimes necessary
Life threatening toxicities	- Discontinue treatment - Dexamethasone

Conclusions

IL-2 is a pleiotropic cytokine, which can cause many side effects upon systemic administration. Although the mechanisms by which IL-2 induces toxicities are not exactly known, release of secondary cytokines, lymphocytic infiltration and oedema due to the VLS can all contribute to the side effects observed during this treatment. These effects cannot be predicted from in vitro studies and only partly from animal models. It is not clear whether separation of anti-tumour efficacy from toxicity is possible, because it is not known which mechanisms are responsible for anti-tumour response.

More studies are required to elucidate these mechanisms in the hope of optimising the clinical use of this cytokine.

References

1. Rosenberg SA, Lotze MJ, Yang JC, et al. Experience with the use of high dose interleukin-2 in the treatment of 652 cancer patients. Ann Surg 1989; 210: 474–85.
2. West WH, Tauer KW, Yanelli JR, et al. Constant-infusion recombinant Interleukin-2 in adoptive immunotherapy of advanced cancer. N Eng J Med 1987; 316: 898–905.
3. Eberlein TJ, Schoof DD, Jung SE, et al. A new regimen of interleukin-2 and lymphokine activated killer cells. Efficacy without significant toxicity. Arch Int Med 1988; 148: 2571–6.

4. Dutcher JP, Creekmore S, Weiss GR, et al. A phase II study of interleukin-2 and lymphokine activated killer cells in patients with metastatic malignant melanoma. J Clin Oncol 1989; 7: 477–85.
5. Fisher RJ, Coltman CA, Doroshow JH. Metastatic renal cell cancer treated with interleukin-2 and lymphokine activated killer cells. Ann Int Med 1988; 108: 518–23.
6. Margolin KA, Rayner AA, Hawkins MJ, et al. Interleukin-2 and lymphokine-activated killer cell therapy of solid tumors: Analysis of toxicty and management guidelines. J Clin Oncol 1989; 7: 486–98.
7. Siegel JP, Puri RK. Interleukin-2 toxicity. J Clin Oncol 1991; 9: 694–704.
8. Atzpodien J, Körfer A, Franks CR, et al. Home therapy with recombinant interleukin-2 and interferon α 2b in advanced human malignancies. Lancet 1990; 335: 1509–12.
9. Mitchell MS, Kempf RA, Harel W, et al. Effectiveness and tolerability of low-dose cyclophosphamide and low dose Intravenous Interleukin-2 in disseminated melanoma. J Clin Oncol 1988; 6: 409–24.
10. Thompson JA, Lee DJ, Lindgren CG, et al. Influence of schedule of Interleukin-2 administration on therapy with Interleukin-2 and lymphokine activated killer cells. Cancer Res 1989; 49: 235–40.
11. Rosenstein M, Ettinghausen SE, Rosenberg SA. Extravasation of intravascular fluid mediated by the systemic administration of recombinant interleukin-2. J Immunol 1986; 137: 1735–42.
12. Mier JW, Vachino G, Van der Meer JW, et al. Induction of circulating tumor necrosis factor (TNF alpha) as the mechanism for the febrile response to interleukin-2 (IL-2) in cancer patients. J Clin Immunol 1988; 8: 426–36.
13. Gemlo BT, Palladino MA, Jaffe HS, et al. Circulating cytokines in patients with metastatic cancer treated with recombinant Interleukin 2 and lymphokine-activated-killer cells. Cancer Res 1988; 48: 5864–67.
14. Kasahara T, Hooks JJ, Daugherty SF, Oppenheim JJ. Interleukin-2 mediated immune interferon (IFN-γ) production by human T cells and T cell subsets. J Immunol 1983; 130: 1784–89.
15. Nedwin GE, Svedersky LP, Bringman TS, et al. Effect of interleukin-2, interferon-g and mitogens on the production of tumor necrosis factors α and β. J Immunol 1985; 135: 2492–7.
16. Marshall ME, Cibull MH, Peason T, et al. Human recombinant Interleukin-2 provokes infiltration of lymphocytes into myocardium and liver in rabbits. J Biol Response Mod 1990; 9: 279–87.
17. Anderson TD, Hayes TJ. Toxicity of human recombinant Interleukin-2 in rats. Pathologic changes are characterized by marked lymphocytic and eosinophilic proliferation and multisystem involvement. Lab Invest 1989; 60: 331–46.
18. Thijs LG, Hack CE, Strack van Schijndel RJM, et al. Activation of the complement system during immunotherapy with Interleukin-2. Relation to the development of side effects. J Immunol 1990; 144: 2419–24.
19. Prozanski W, Vadas P. Phospholipase A2 – a mediator between proximal and distal effectors of inflammation. Immunol Today 1991; 12: 143–6.
20. Ettinghausen SE, Puri RK, Rosenberg SA. Increased vascular permeability in organs mediated by the systemic administration of lymphokine-activated killer cells and recombinant Interleukin-2 in Mice. J Natl Cancer Inst 1988; 80: 177–88.
21. Fairman RP, Glauser FL, Merchant RE, et al. Increase of rat pulmonary microvascular permeability to albumin by recombinant interleukin-2. Cancer Res 1987; 47: 3528–32.
22. Anderson TD, Hayes TJ, Gately MK, et al. Toxicity of human recombinant Interleukin-2 in the mouse is mediated by Interleukin-activated lymphocytes. Separation of efficacy and toxicity by selective lymphocyte subset depletion. Lab Invest 1988; 59: 598–612.
23. Aronson FR, Libby P, Brandon EP, et al. IL-2 rapidly induces natural killer adhesion to human endothelial cells. A potential mechanism for endothelial injury. J Immunol 1988; 141: 158–63.
24. Damle NK, Doyle LV. IL-2 activated human killer lymphocytes but not their secreted products

mediate increase in albumin flux across cultured endothelial Monolayers. Implication for vascular leak syndrome. J Immunol 1989; 142: 2660.
25. Ferro TJ, Johnson A, Everitt J, Malik AB. IL-2 induces pulmonary edema and vasoconstruction independent of circulating lymphocytes. J Immunol 1989; 142: 1916–21.
26. Beckhard DE, Fairman RP, Hinshaw DB, et al. In vivo Interleukin-2 activated sheep lung lymph lymphocytes increase ovine vascular endothelial permeability by non-lytic mechanisms. Eur J Cancer 1990; 26: 1074–8.
27. Cotran RS, Pober JS, Gimbrone MA Jr, et al. Endothelial activation during interleukin-2 immunotherapy. A possible mechanism for the vascular leak syndrome. J Immunol 1988; 140: 1883–8.
28. Stolpen AH, Guinan EC, Fiers W, et al. Recombinant tumor necrosis factor and immune interferon act simply and in combination to reorganize human vascular endothelial cell monolayers. Am J Pathol 1986; 123: 16–24.
29. Puri RK, Rosenberg SA. Combined effects of interferon α and interleukin 2 on the induction of a vascular leak syndrome in mice. Cancer Immunol Immunother 1989; 28: 267–74.
30. Mier JW, Brandon EP, Libby P, et al. Activated endothelial cells resist lymphokine-activated killer cell-mediated injury: possible role of induced cytokines in limiting capillary leak during IL-2 therapy. J Immunol 1989; 143: 2407–14.
31. Puri RK, Travis WD, Rosenberg SA. Decrease in Interleukin-2 induced vascular leakage in the lungs of mice by administration of recombinant Interleukin 1α in vivo. Cancer Res 1989; 49: 969–76.
32. Baars JW, Hack CE, Wagstaff J, et al. The activation of polymorphonuclear neutrophils and the complement system during immunotherapy with recombinant interleukin-2. Br J Cancer 1992; 65: 96–101.
33. Vachino G, Gelfand JA, Atkins MB, et al. Complement activation in cancer patients undergoing immunotherapy with interleukin-2 (IL-2): binding of complement and C-reactive protein by IL-2 activated lymphocytes. Blood 1991; 78: 2505–13.
34. Welbourn R, Goldman G, Kobzik L, et al. Involvement of thromboxane and neutrophils in multiple-system organ edema with interleukin-2. Ann Surg 1990; 212: 728–33.
35. Slotman GJ, Burchard KW, Williams JJ, et al. Interaction of prostaglandins, activated complement and granulocytes in clinical sepsis and hypotension. Surgery 1986; 90: 744–54.
36. Lee RE, Lotze MT, Skibber JM, et al. Cardiorespiratory effects of immunotherapy with Interleukin-2. J Clin Oncol 1989; 7:7–20.
37. Ognibene FP, Rosenberg SA, Lotze M, et al. Interleukin-2 administration causes reversible hemodynamic changes and left ventricular dysfunction similar to those seen in septic shock. Chest 1988; 94: 750–4.
38. Davis SD, Berkmen YM, Wang JCL. Interleukin-2 therapy for advanced renal cell carcinoma: Radiographic evaluation of response and complications. Radiology 1990; 177: 127–31.
39. Gaynor ER, Vitek L, Sticklin L, et al. The hemodynamic efects of treatment with Interleukin-2 and lymphokine activated killer cells. Ann Int Med 1988; 109: 953–8.
40. Nora R, Abrams JS, Tait NC, et al. Myocardial toxic effects during recombinant Interleukin-2 therapy. J Natl Cancer Inst 1989; 81: 59–63.
41. Osanto S, Cluitmans FRM, Franks CR, et al. Myocardial injury after interleukin-2 therapy. Lancet 1988; 11: 48–9(Letter to the editor).
42. Sobotka PA, McMannis J, Fisher RI, et al. Effect of Interleukin-2 or cardiac function in the isolated rat heart. J Clin Invest 1990; 86: 845–50.
43. Favalli L, Lanza E, Rozza A, et al. Evaluation of the cardiovascular toxic effect of recombinant Interleukin-2 in Rats. Anticancer Res 1990; 10: 1693–8.
44. Gulick T, Chung MK, Pieper SJ, et al. Interleukin 1 and tumor necrosis factor inhibit cardiac myocyte beta-adrenergic responsiveness. Proc Natl Acad Sci USA 1986; 86: 6753–7.
45. Hanis RL, Musker DM, Bloom K, et al. Manifestations of sepsis. Arch Int Med 1987; 147: 1895–906.
46. Glauser MP, Zanetti G, Baumgartner JD, Cohen J. Septic shock: pathogenesis. Lancet 1991; 338: 732–6.

47. Nuyens JH, Huybregts CCM, Eerenberg-Belmer AJM, et al. Quantification of plasma factor XIIa-C1 inhibitor and Kallikrein-C1 inhibitor complexes in sepsis. Blood 1988; 72: 1841–8.
48. Hack CE, Wagstaff J, Strack van Schijndel RJM, et al. Studies on the contact system of coagulation during therapy with high dose of recombinant IL-2: Implications for septic shock. Thromb Haemost 1991; 65: 497–504.
49. Jacobs HS, Craddock PR, Hammerschimdt DE, Moldow CF. Complement induced granulocyte aggregation. N Engl J Med 1980; 302: 789–94.
50. Kilbourn RG, Belloni P. Endothelial cell production of nitrogen oxides in response to Interferon g in combination with tumor necrosis factor, Interleukin-1 or Endotoxin. J Natl Cancer Inst 1990; 82: 772–6.
51. Nathan CF, Stuehr DJ. Does endothelium-derived nitric oxide have a role in cytokine-induced hypotension? J Natl Cancer Inst 1990; 82: 726–8.(Editorial)
52. Kilbourn RG, Jubran A, Gross SS, et al. Reversal of endotoxin-mediated shock by N^G-methyl-L-arginine, an inhibitor of nitric oxide synthesis. Bioch Biophys Res Commun 1990; 172: 1132–8.
53. Hibbs JB, Westenfelder C, Taintor R, et al. Evidence for cytokine-inducible nitric oxide synthesis from L-arginine in patients receiving interleukin-2 therapy. J Clin Invest 1992; 89: 867–77.
54. Harms BA, Pahl AC, Pohlman, et al. Effects of interleukin-2 on pulmonary and systemic transvascular fluid filtration. Surgery 1989; 106: 339–46.
55. Glauser FL, de Blois GG, Bechard E, et al. Cardiopulmonary effects of recombinant interleukin-2 infusion in sheep. J Appl Physiol 1988; 64: 1030–7.
56. Butler LD, Mohler KM, Layman NK, et al. Interleukin-2 induced systemic toxicity: induction of mediators and immunopharmacologic intervention. Immunopharm Immunotox 1989; 11: 445–87.
57. Klausner JM, Paterson IS, Morel NML, et al. Role of thomboxane in Interleukin 2 induced lung injury in sheep. Cancer Res 1989; 49: 3542–9.
58. Textor SC, Margolin K, Blayney D, et al. Renal, volume, and hormonal changes during therapeutic administration of recombinant interleukin-2 in man. Am J Med 1987; 83: 1055–61.
59. Webb DE, Austin HA III, Belldegrun A, et al. Metabolic and renal effects of interleukin-2 immunotherapy for metastatic cancer. Clin Nephrol 1988; 30: 141–5.
60. Kozeny GA, Nicolas JD, Creekmore S, et al. Effects of Interleukin-2 immunotherapy on renal function. J Clin Oncol 1988; 6: 1170–6.
61. Shalmi CL, Dutcher JP, Feinfeld DA, et al. Acute renal dysfunction during interleukin-2 treatment. Suggestion of an intrinsic renal lesion. J Clin Oncol 1990; 8: 1839–46.
62. Belldegrun A, Webb DE, Austin HA III, et al. Renal toxicity of Interleukin-2 administration in patients with metastatic renal cell cancer: effect of pre-therapy nephrectomy. J Urol 1989; 141: 499–503.
63. Sosman JA, Kohler PC, Hank JA, et al. Repetitive weekly cycles of interleukin-2. Clinical and immunologic effects of dose, schedule, and addition of indomethacin. J Natl Cancer Inst. 1988; 80: 1451–61.
64. Schwartzentruber D, Lotze MT, Rosenberg SA. Colonic perforation. An unusual complication of therapy with high-dose Interleukin-2. Cancer 1988; 62: 2350–3.
65. Birchfield GR, Ward JH, Redman BG, et al. Interleukin-2 immunotherapy for malignant melanoma. West J Med 1990; 152: 714–6.
66. Fisher B, Keenan AM, Garra BS, et al. Interleukin-2 induces profound reversible cholestasis: A detailed analysis in treated cancer patients. J Clin Oncol 1989; 7: 1852–62.
67. Jablons DM, Mule JM, McIntosh J, et al. Interleukin 6/Interferon-β2 as a circulating hormone: Induction by cytokine administration in humans. J Immunol 1989; 142: 1542–7.
68. Imura H, Fukata J, Mori T. Cytokines and endocrine function: an interaction between the immune and neuroendocrine systems. Clinical Endocrinol 1991; 35: 107–15.
69. Atkins MB, Mier JW, Parkinson DR, et al. Hypothyroidism after treatment with interleukin-2 and lymphokine-activated killer cells. N Eng J Med 1988; 318: 1557–63.

70. Van Liessum PA, de Mulder PHM, Mattijssen EJM, et al. Hypothyroidism and goitre during interleukin-2 therapy without LAK cells. Lancet 1989; ii: 224(Letter).
71. Burman P, Tötterman TH, Oberg K, Karlsson FA. Thyroid auto-immunity in patients on long term therapy with leucocyte-derived Interferon. J Clin Endocrinol Metab 1986; 63: 1086–90.
72. Fentiman IS, Balkwill FR, Thomas BS, et al. An autoimmune actiology for hypothyroidism following Interferon therapy for breast cancer. Eur J Cancer Clin Oncol 1988; 24: 1299–303.
73. Weetman AP, Volkman DJ, Burman KD, et al. The in vitro regulation of human thyrocyte HLA-DR antigen expression. J Clin Endocrin Metab 1985; 61: 817–24.
74. Martin A, Huber GK, Davies TF. Induction of human thyroid cell ICAM-1 (CD-54) antigen expression and ICAM-1 mediated lymphocyte binding. Endocrinology 1990; 127: 651–7.
75. Kung AWC, Jones BM, Lai CL. Effects of interferon-γ therapy on thyroid function, T-lymphocyte subpopulations and induction of autoantibodies. J Endocrinol Metab 1990; 71: 1230–4.
76. Bogner U, Single B, Schleusener H. Interferon-γ protects human thyroid epithelial cells against cell mediated cytotoxicity. Immunobiol 1988; 176: 423–31.
77. Hoekman K, Von Blomberg-van de Flier BME, Wagstaff J, et al. Reversible thyroid dysfunction during treatment with GM-CSF. Lancet 1991; 338: 541–2.
78. Schaafsma MR, Falkenburg JHF, Landegent JE, et al. In vivo production of interleukin-5, granulocyte-macrophage colony-stimulating factor, macrophage-colony-stimulating factor and interleukin-6 during intravenous administration of high dose interleukin-2 in cancer patients. Blood 1991; 78: 1981–87.
79. Michie HR, Eberlein TJ, Spriggs DR, et al. Interleukin-2 initiates metabolic responses associated with critical illness in humans. Ann Surg 1988; 208: 493–501.
80. Atkins MB, Gould JA, Allegretta M, et al. Phase I evaluation of recombinant interleukin-2 in patients with advanced malignant disease. J Clin Oncol 1986; 4: 1380–91.
81. Denicoff KD, Durkin TM, Lotze MT, et al. The neuroendocrine effects of interleukin-2 treatment. J Clin Endocrinol Metab 1989; 69: 402–20.
82. Vetto JT, Papa MZ, Lotze MT, et al. Reduction of toxicity of interleukin-2 and lymphokine-activated killer cells in humans by the administration of corticosteroids. J Clin Oncol 1987; 5: 496–503.
83. Van der Molen LA, Smith JWII, Longo DL, et al. Adrenal insufficiency and Interleukin-2 therapy. Ann Intern Med 1989; 111: 185(Letter).
84. Wilson DE, Birchfield GR, Hejazi JS, et al. Hypocholesterolemia in patients treated with recombinant Interleukin-2. Appearance of remnant-like lipoprotein. J Clin Oncol 1989; 7: 1573–8.
85. Gaspari AA, Lotze MT, Rosenberg SA, et al. Dermatologic changes associated with Interleukin-2 administration. JAMA 1987; 258: 1624–9.
86. Weinstein A, Brijak D, Mittelman A, et al. Erythema nodosum in a patients with renal cell carcinoma treated with interleukin-2 and lymphokine-activated killer cells. JAMA 1987; 258: 3120–1.
87. Mier JW, Aronson FR, Numer of PR, et al. Toxicity of immunotherapy with interleukin-2 and lymphokine-activated killer cells. Path Immunopathol Res 1988; 7: 459–76.
88. Ramseur WL, Richards FII, Duggan DB. A case of fatal pemphigus vulgaris in association with beta interferon and interleukin-2 therapy. Cancer 1989; 63: 2005–7.
89. Staunton MR, Sailly MC, Le Boit PE, Aronson FR. Life threatening bullous skin eruptions during Interleukin-2 therapy. J Natl Cancer Inst 1991; 83: 56–7.
90. Lee RE, Gaspari AA, Lotze MT, et al. Interleukin-2 and psoriasis. Arch Dermatol 1988; 124: 1811–5.
91. Denicoff KD, Rubinow DR, Papa MZ. The neuropsychiatric effects of treatment with Interleukin-2 and lymphokine-activated killer cells. Ann Int Med 1987; 107: 293–300.
92. Ellison MD, Povlishock JT, Merchant RE. Blood-brain barried dysfunction in cats following recombinant Interleukin-2 infusion. Cancer Res 1987; 47: 5765–70.
93. Parkinson DR. Interleukin-2 in cancer therapy. Semin Oncol 1988; 15: 10–26.

94. Goey SH, Voerman HJ, Strack van Schijndel RJM, et al. Swelling of metastatic tumors with high-dose interleukin therapy. N Engl J Med 1988; 318: 643–4(Letter).
95. Ettinghausen SE, Moore JG, White DE, et al. Hematologic effects of immunotherapy with lymphokine-activated killer cells and recombinant Interleukin-2 in cancer patients. Blood 1987; 69: 1654–60.
96. Tritarelli E, Rocca E, Testa U, et al. Adoptive immunotherapy with high dose interleukin-2: kinetics of circulating progenitors correlate with interleukin-6. Blood 1991; 77: 741–9.
97. Enokihara H, Furusawa S, Nakakubo H, et al. T cells from eosinophilic patients produce Interleukin-5 with Interleukin-2 stimulation. Blood 1989; 73: 1809–13.
98. Perez R, Padavic K, Krigel R, Weiner L. Antierythrocyte autoantibody formation after therapy with Interleukin-2 and Gamma-Interferon. Cancer 1991; 67: 2512–7.
99. Nawroth PP, Stern DM. Tumor necrosis factor/cachectin-induced modulation of endothelial cell hemostatic properties. Onkologie 1987; 10: 254–8.
100. Van der Poll T, Buller HR, ten Cate H, et al. Activation of coagulation after administration of tumor necrosis factor to normal subjects. N Eng J Med 1990; 332: 1622–7.
101. Suffredini AF, Harpel PC, Parillo JE. Promotion and subsequent inhibition of plasminogen activation after administration of intravenous endotoxin to normal subjects. N Engl J Med 1989; 320: 165–1172.
102. Richard V, Bernier M, Themelin L, et al. Blood coagulation abnormalities during adoptive immunotherapy with interleukin-2 (r Met Hu IL-2 [ala125]). Ann Oncol 1991; 2: 67–8.
103. Kahalek MB, Le Roy EC. Interleukin-2 in scleroderma: correlation of serum level with extent of skin involvement and disease duration. Ann Intern Med 1989; 110: 446–50.
104. Hooks JJ, Moutsopaulos HM, Geis SA, et al. Immune interferon in the circulation of patients with autoimmune disease. N Eng J Med 1979; 301: 5–8.
105. Jones AL, Cropley I, O'Brien MER, et al. Infectious complications of subcutaneous interleukin-2 and interferon-alpha. Lancet 1992; 339: 181–2.
106. Bock SN, Lee RE, Fisher B, et al. A prospective randomzied trial evaluating prophylactic antibiotics to prevent triple-lumen catheter-related sepsis in patients treated with immunotherapy. J Clin Oncol 1990; 8: 161–9.
107. Hardy JR, Moore J, Lorentzos A, et al. Infectious complications of interleukin-2 therapy. Cytokine 1990; 2: 311.
108. Murphy PM, Lane HC, Gallin JL, et al. Marked disparity in incidence of bacterial infections in patients with the acquired immuno-deficiency syndrome receiving interleukin-2 or interferon-alpha. Ann Intern Med 1988; 108: 36–41.
109. Wiebke EA, Rosenberg SA, Lotze MT. Acute immunologic effects of interleukin-2 therapy in cancer patients. Decreased delayed type hypersensitivity response and decreased proliferative response to soluble antigens. J Clin Oncol 1988; 6: 1440–9.
110. Jabbons D, Bolton E, Mertin S, et al. Interleukin-2 based immunotherapy alters circulating neutrophils Fc receptor expression and chemotoxis. J Immunol 1990; 144: 3630–6.
111. Klempner MS, Noring R, Mier JW, et al. An acquired chemotactic defect in neutrophils from patients receiving interleukin-2 immunotherapy. N Eng J Med 1990; 332: 959–66.
112. Balkwill FR. Abnormal IL-2 production and IL-2 receptor expression in haematological malignancies. (Resp: understanding the role of cytokines in the process of malignancy) In: Balkwill FR, editor. Cytokines in cancer therapy. Oxford: Oxford University Press, 1989: 110–3 (resp. 238-9).
113. Mavligit GM, Zakiwiski A, Gutterman JU, et al. Splenic versus hepatic artery infusion of Interleukin-2 in patients with liver metastases. J Clin Oncol 1990; 8: 319–24.
114. Eggermont AMM, Goey SH, Wiggers TH, et al. Hepatic artery infusion with Interleukin-2 in patients with unresectable colorectal hepatic metastatic disease: A phase 1B Study. Nat Immun Cell Growth Regul 1990; 9: 73–4.
115. Steis RG, Urba WJ, Van der Molen LA, et al. Intraperitoneal lymphokine-activated killer cell and Interleukin-2 therapy for malignancies limited to the peritoneal cavity. J Clin Oncol 1990; 8: 1618–29.

116. Yasumoto K, Miyuzaki K, Nagaskima A, et al. Induction of lymphokine-activated killer cells by intrapleural instillations of recombinant interleukin-2 in patients with malignant pleurisy due to lung cancer. Cancer Res 1987; 47: 2184–7.
117. Eggermont AMM, Goey SH, Slingerland R, et al. Intrapleural administration of recombinant Interleukin-2 (IL-2) in patients with malignant pleural mesothelioma: A Phase II study. Nat Immun Cell Growth Regul 1990; 9: 74–5(abstract).
118. Blancher A, Roubinet F, Grancher AS, et al. Adoptive local immunotherapy of malignant gliomas. Nat Immun Cell Growth Regul 1990; 9: 72(abstract).
119. Merchant RE, Ellison MD, Young HF. Immunotherapy for malignant glioma using human recombinant interleukin-2 and activated autologous lymphocytes. A review of preclinical and clinical investigations. J Neuro Oncol 1990; 8: 173–88.
120. Hulan E, Hulan H. Local continuous high dose Interleukin-2: a new therapeutic model for the treatment of advanced bladder carcinoma. Cancer Res 1989; 49: 5469–74.
121. Kolitz JE, Wong GY, Welte K, et al. Phase I trial of recombinant interleukin-2 and cyclophosphamide. Augmentation of cellular immunity and T-cell mitogenic response with long-term administration of r IL-2. J Biol Response Mod 1988; 7: 457–72.
122. Kirchner H, Körfer A, Evers P, et al. The development of neutralizing antibodies in a patient receiving subcutaneous recombinant and natural Interleukin-2. Cancer 1991; 67: 1862–4.
123. Mule JJ, Shu S, Schwarz SL, et al. Adoptive immunotherapy of established pulmonary metastases with LAK cells and recombinant interleukin-2. Science 1984; 225: 1487–9.
124. La Freniere R, Rosenberg SA. Successful immunotherapy of murine experimental hepatic metastases with lymphokine-activated killer cells and recombinant interleukin-2. Cancer Res 1985; 45: 3735–41.
125. Weiss GR, Margolin KA, Aronson FR, et al. A randomized phase II trial of continuous infusion interleukin-2 or bolus injection interleukin-2 plus lymphokine-activated killer cells for advanced renal cell carcinoma. J Clin Oncol 1992; 10: 275–81.
126. Silagi S, Schaefer AE. Successful immunotherapy of mouse melanoma and sarcoma with recombinant Interleukin-2 and Cyclophosphamide. J Biol Response Mod 1986; 5: 411–22.
127. Papa MZ, Yang JC, Vetto JC, et al. Combined effects of chemotherapy and interleukin-2 in the therapy of mice with advanced pulmonary tumors. Cancer Res 1988; 48: 122–9.
128. Lindeman A, Höffner K, Schmidt RE, et al. A phase II study of low dose cyclophosphamide and recombinant human interleukin-2 in metastatic renal cell carcinoma and malignant melanoma. Cancer Immunol Immunother 1989; 28: 275–81.
129. Mier JW, Vachino G, Klempner M, et al. Inhibition of Interleukin-2-induced tumor necrosis factor release by dexamethasone: prevention of an acquired neutrophil chematoxis defect and differential suppression of Interleukin-2 associated side effects. Blood 1990; 76: 1933–40.
130. Fraker DL, Langstein HN, Norton JA. Passive immunization against tumor necrosis factor partially abrogates interleukin-2 toxicity. J Exp Med 1989; 170: 1015–20.
131. Blay JY, Favrot MC, Negrier S, et al. Correlation between clinical response to Interleukin-2 therapy and sustained production of tumor necrosis factor. Cancer Res 1990; 50: 2371–4.
132. Schwartzberg L, Tauer K, Birch R, et al. Phase I study of sequential recombinant tumor necrosis factor (rTNF) and recombinant interleukin-2 (r-IL-2) in patients with advanced malignancy. Proc ASCO 1989; 8: 183(abstract).
133. Baars JW, de Boer JP, Wagstaff J, et al. Interleukin-2 induces activation and fibrinolysis: resemblance to changes seen during experimental endotoxaemia. BJ Haematol. 1992; 82: 285–301.

5. Interleukin-2 biology and immunology

GIORGIO PARMIANI and CARLO GAMBACORTI-PASSERINI

Biology of interleukin-2

Interleukin-2 (IL-2), formerly known as T Cell growth factor, is a 15 KD inducible glycoprotein synthesized by T lymphocytes and plays a pivotal role in the lymphocyte activation network. In particular, IL-2 represents the most important growth factor for T lymphocytes and NK cells.

Structure/function of IL-2

The IL-2 gene, which is located in humans on chromosome 4q [1], contains four exons and codes for a polypetide of 153 aminoacids. This precursor protein is then processed inside the cell to the mature form of 133 aminoacids, by the removal of the first 20 amino-terminal residues and is finally secreted. The mature IL-2 contains one disulphide bridge between two cysteines at position 58 and 105 [2, 3]. A third cysteine residue is located at position 125 and is not normally involved in intramolecular bridges. However, this residue can react with another 125Cys on a different IL-2 molecule, thus forming a dimer that is biologically inactive. For this reason, many IL-2 cDNAs have been mutagenized at position 125.

In 1983, Taniguchi and co-workers cloned the human IL-2 gene [4]. The cDNA coding for the mature form of IL-2 was subsequently inserted and expressed in eukaryotic and in prokaryotic vectors [5]. However, the IL-2 polypeptide undergoes minor post-translational modifications in maturation which have little if any impact on its biological activity [3]. The recombinant IL-2 (rIL-2) molecules made in *E. Coli* or in other bacterial vectors are, therefore, likely to have the same activity as natural IL-2.

The availability of large quantities of IL-2 made it possible to obtain crystals of IL-2 and, therefore, to study the three dimensional structure by X-ray crystallography [6]. IL-2 was discovered to be an α-helical protein (Figure 1). It has several helical segments interrupted by extended loops containing proline residues. There are no segments of β secondary structure in the molecule. Current data suggest that IL-2 binds two/three receptor molecules, with two

J. Wagstaff (ed.), The Role of Interleukin-2 in the Treatment of Cancer Patients, 71-83.

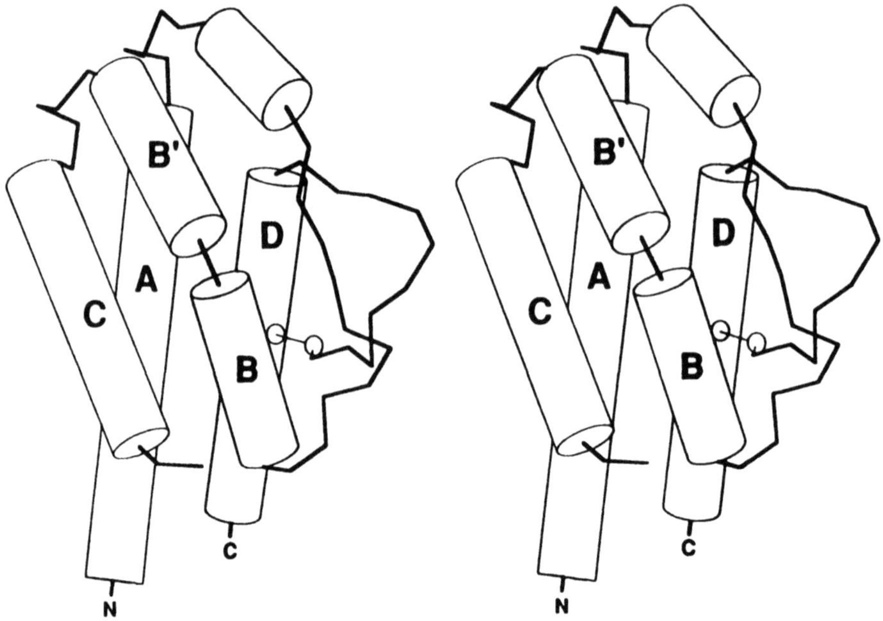

Figure 1. (A) Cα atom backbone trace of one [Ala^{125}]IL-2 molecule. (B) Schematic drawing of [Ala^{125}]IL-2; helices are shown as cylinders; picture produced by a program written by A.M. Lesk and K.D. Hardman. Disulfide is shown in both figures. (From McKay B. et al., Science, 1992, 257, 412-413, with permission.)

independent binding sites. Antibodies to peptides that react with different parts of the IL-2 molecule have been used to map global regions in the IL-2 sequence likely to be important in receptor binding [7, 8]. These data also indicate that residues involved in binding to either the p55 or the p70 receptor subunit map to two contiguous patches on the surface of human IL-2 structure (Zurawski SM et al., unpublished).

Interaction of IL-2 with its receptor

IL-2 delivers its growth signal by virtue of its interaction with a specific cell surface receptor. Recent studies suggest that the IL-2 receptor (IL-2R) is composed of at least three chains [9]. One (α chain or p55) binds IL-2 with low affinity (Kd = 10 nM) and does not transduce any signal by itself. It is not expressed on resting leukocytes but appears on the membranes of T and B lymphocytes following initial activation [10]. A second molecule (β chain or p75) is constitutively expressed by a small proportion (5-15%) of peripheral blood lymphocytes, embracing all CD16+ cells, and less than 5% of T and B lymphocytes [11]. p75 binds IL-2 with intermediate affinity (Kd = 1 nM) and seems to transduce a signal into the cell. It is not, however, known whether the capability for signal transduction is possessed by p75 on its own, or instead is a property of the complex between p75 and a third (γ) chain of the IL-2 receptor [9]. About 5% of p55 molecules on the cell membrane interact via non-covalent forces with p75 to create a receptor that binds IL-2 with very high affinity (Kd = 10 pM). IL-2 binds rapidly to the receptor by interacting with p55. It is then tightly held by an interaction with the binding site on p75. The γ chain, which has been recently discovered [12, 13], cannot bind IL-2 but seems necessary for signal transduction.

p55 (also named CD25) is readily shed from lymphocyte membranes into extracellular fluids and can be measured in the serum, especially after immune responses. However, given the low affinity of CD25 for IL-2, it is improbable that soluble CD25 can effectively compete with cellular receptors for the available IL-2 [14].

Signal transduction

It is known that IL-2, upon interaction with its receptor, is able to transduce an intracellular signal culminating in the entry of the cell into the S phase. The biochemical nature of the initial nuclear signaling mechanism has not been elucidated. Increasing evidence suggests, however, that tyrosine protein kinases and serine/threonine protein kinases may be involved in the IL-2-dependent proliferative signals [15-17]. As none of the known components of the IL-2R (p55 and p75) has been shown to possess detectable kinase activity, it is likely that enzymes distinct from the identified IL-2R chains play roles in signal transduction.

It has been recently shown that IL-2, through the binding to its receptor can induce the phosphorylation of one of the most abundant T-cell tyrosine phosphokinases, $p56^{lck}$ [18]. It has also been reported that IL-2 can induce phosphorylation and activation of a serine/threonine kinase called p72-74 encoded by the c-Raf-1 protooncogene [19], a kinase which has been recently implicated in signal-transduction events mediated by several tyrosine kinase growth factor receptors and oncogene products [20]. The relationship of these kinases with the γ chain of the IL-2R is still obscure.

Cellular distribution of the IL-2R

Although IL-2R are most commonly expressed on the membrane of T lymphocytes and NK cells [10, 11], other cell types have been shown to possess IL-2R. B lymphocytes and monocytes possess functional IL-2R, but also epidermal Langherans cells and oligodendrocytes can be stimulated by IL-2 to proliferate [21-24] and, in the case of oligodendroglial cells, to express the myelin basic protein messenger RNA [25].

IL-2R have also been occasionally described to be expressed on melanoma cells, chronic lymphocytic leukemia (CLL), acute myeloid and acute lymphoblastic leukemia cells [26-29]. However, with the exception of CLL, it is not clear whether IL-2R are functional in these cases and whether they can impart a mitogenic signal in vivo. Moreover, under physiological conditions, IL-2 is released locally during an active immune response (see below) and, therefore, systemic IL-2 levels are usually very low (0.5 U/ml) or absent. This fact is also explained by the rapid distribution and clearance of IL-2 from the body, with initial half lives for injected doses of IL-2 in the order of few minutes [30].

Immunology

IL-2 has a central role in immunology due to its ability to trigger and regulate the proliferation, differentiation and functional activation of important immune cells like NK, T and B lymphocytes and macrophages [10]. In particular, IL-2 has a basic function in the growth of circulating T lymphocytes that have recognized the nominal antigen with their T-cell receptor (TCR). In fact, only a limited number of T lymphocytes can recognize a given antigen and IL-2 appears instrumental in stimulating the expansion of such clones through their IL-2R and to ensure that an appropriate immune response will take place. These lymphocyte precursors need to go through several differentiation steps and rounds of division which all require the presence of IL-2 before other cytokines, like IL-4 and IFN-γ can activate specific programs of differentiation.

Mitogenic effect on T, NK and B cells

Interaction of TCR with the nominal antigen leads to proliferation and to transcriptional activation of both the IL-2 gene and the gene encoding IL-2R [31]. The binding of IL-2R by IL-2 results in a further mitogenic signal. The presence of IL-2, therefore, enables T cells to activate a complex program of proliferation and differentiation toward a functional active state. The mitogenic effect thus will depend both on the IL-2 concentration and on the expression of high affinity IL-2 R which in turn will depend on the specific antigenic stimulation. The interplay of these three main factors determines the time and magnitude of the mitogenic effect and T cell expansion [10]. It is evident that a balance between occupation of high affinity IL-2R by IL-2 and their de novo synthesis induced by the TCR-mediated antigen recognition will establish whether or not T cells will return to the resting stage in which no high affinity IL-2R are expressed and cells cannot be further stimulated unless a new TCR-antigen interaction will again induce the expression of IL-2R. It should be noted, however, that a small subset of CD3+, CD8+, CD11b+ T cells has been identified which respond to IL-2 in the absence of antigens and generates cells with lymphokine-activated killer (LAK) activity [32]. In the presence of accessory cells, however, even resting T cells can develop LAK activity [33]. Recently, IL-2 has been shown to play an important role even in the programmed cell death (apoptosis) of T cells. In fact, IL-2 has been reported to be a critical determinant in driving both CD4+ and CD8+ T cells to apoptosis which ensues when T cells encounter the antigen which binds to their TCR after IL-2 exposure [34].

The presence of IL-2, either physiologically produced by T cells or artificially added in vitro, is also necessary to trigger the proliferation of NK cells defined as TCR-, CD3-, CD16+ and/or CD56+ lymphocytes [35]. In fact, IL-2 causes proliferation of mature NK cells through their constitutive expression of IL-2Rβ chain (p75) with intermediate affinity [36], as shown by the inhibition of proliferation occurring in the presence of anti-IL-2Rβ antibodies [11]. In addition, IL-2 induces a prompt IL-2Rα (p55) synthesis by human, but not murine, NK cells [37].

IL-2 mitogenic effect on NK cells can be increased or reduced by a variety of other cytokines. It is worth mentioning the recently described NK cell stimulatory factor (NKCSF), a heterodimeric cytokine produced by B-cell lines and which potentiates the IL-2 effect although by itself is unable to stimulate NK proliferation [38]. IL-7, but not IL-6 [39], by itself is able to trigger proliferation of resting NK cells but when a suboptimal dose of IL-2 is used, both IL-6 and IL-7 can synergize with IL-2 to increase its mitogenic effect [40]. Cytokines which may block or impair the mitogenic effect of IL-2 on NK cells include IFN-α/β [41] and IL-4 [42]. This complex interaction among different cytokines must be kept in mind when designing clinical protocols in particular when empirical combinations of cytokines (e.g. IL-2/IFNs) are used in order to avoid negative results which might have been predicted by consideration of the above data. In addition to IL-2 and IL-2R, other genes are activated upon interaction of IL-2 with its receptors and internalization of the complex. For example, both T and NK cells will express tumour necrosis factor (TNF)-R which, through the TNF produced endogenously, can help in the generation of LAK activity [43, 44].

Since IL-2 has been widely used in the immunotherapy of cancer, it is important to understand whether the in vitro studies of mitogenic effect of IL-2 on T and NK cells reflect a phenomenon which also occurs in vivo. There is ample evidence that antigenic-specific T cells can be grown in vivo for long period of time upon administration of IL-2 and antigens [45], a feature which offers an important rationale for using tumour-specific T cells and IL-2 in adoptive immunotherapy of human tumours. CD8+, tumour-specific CTL clones or lines also survive and cause regression of established metastases in mice given such lymphocyte lines along with non-toxic doses of IL-2 [46].

Even NK cells can be expanded in vivo by IL-2 although in the mouse, and at variance with T cells, NK are not induced to express the p55 IL-2α gene [47]. In the cancer patients treated with IL-2, NK cells were reported to increase and proliferate [48] although such evidence, as assessed by examining CD16+ cells in the peripheral blood, has not been obtained in other studies [49].

Less documentation relates to the expansion of B cells exposed to IL-2 both in vitro and in vivo since the effect of IL-2 on these lymphocytes appears to be confined to differentiation and immunoglobulin switch, as shown by studying mice rendered IL-2 deficient by gene targeting [50].

Differentiation and activation of lymphocytes and monocytes

Once IL-2 has triggered the mitogenic programme of T cells, other cytokines are necessary to cause further differentiation of CD4+ and CD8+ T cells (both equally activated by antigen with or without the help of antigen presenting cells) into a more specific functional state [51]. The most important of such cytokines are not only IL-4, IFN-γ and TGF-β [51] but also IL-6 and IL-7 which can play a role in the regulation of different pathways of T cell differentiation toward a fully functional stage [52, 53]. Monocytes can also express IL-2R [22], and such cells can be activated to become tumouricidal after exposure to IL-2 [54]. As has been discussed above, even NK cells are likely to require other factors (such as NKCSF and IFN) in addition to IL-2 to proceed to a fully activated state.

Activation of both T and NK lymphocytes results in two main functions, namely cytotoxicity (and help for T cells) and cytokine production which are by no means mutually exclusive. IL-2 provides both types of activation upon interaction with its receptors on CTL and NK cells. In addition, IL-2 can affect the pathways of thymocyte maturation in vivo [55] since blocking both with anti-IL-2 or anti-IL-2R antibodies in vivo prevents the development of mature, functional T cells and of antigen-specific CTL [56].

The most relevant function induced by IL-2 stimulation both in T and NK cells is cytotoxicity. Although purified resting T cells are usually not stimulated to become cytotoxic by IL-2 alone due to the lack of IL-2R expression in the majority of such cells, a small subpopulation of CD3+, CD8+ lymphocytes have been reported to develop into lytic effectors [32]. T cells obtained from peripheral blood lymphocytes or from tumour lesions and cultured in the presence of large amount of IL-2 (600-6000 IU/ml) expand several hundred or even thousand fold and become lytic against a variety of tumour cell lines. Such a T/LAK activity is, however, usually MHC-unrestricted when T cells are stimulated in the absence of the putative antigen, i.e. autologous tumour cells, and defines a population of T effectors whose role in cancer therapy is still unclear [57]. In fact, the purity of these T cell populations has not usually been adequately evaluated and the presence of a few NK and/or accessory cells which may help in activating T cells cannot be completely ruled out. The cytotoxic potential of T cells but not of NK cells and the gene expression of pore-forming proteins by IL-2 can be significantly increased by IL-6 [58] whereas IL-10 augmented the IL-2 generated cytolytic activity of T cells [59] pointing out again that IL-2 often synergizes with other cytokines in modulating lymphocyte functions.

IL-2 also triggers the lytic activity of NK cells. It has been shown that purified NK cells are stimulated to become cytotoxic against many targets due to their expression of IL-2Rβ even during the resting phase [see 35]. NK cells recognize target cells through an unknown mechanism although there is a distinct possibility that such lymphocytes may use different receptors to recognize tumour cells and to deliver different cytotoxicity signals [60]. After interacting with target cells, NK cells become inactivated but they can recycle again into lytic effectors upon re-exposure to IL-2 [61]. In addition to IL-2, other cytokines such as IFN-α, β and NKCSF enhance spontaneous NK cytotoxicity, but possibly by different mechanisms [35]. IFN-α and -β may however also reduce the cytotoxicity of CD3- cells [62]. NK cells activated by IL-2 have been operationally designated as LAK and, although this definition was originally proposed to account for tumour cytotoxicity developed in vitro by bulk peripheral blood lymphocytes [63], today we know that by and large the majority of the tumour cytotoxic LAK activity is due to NK cells [64].

In vivo administration of IL-2 has been shown to cause phenotypic activation of both T and NK lymphocytes, as evaluated by the increased expression of p55 (CD25) IL-2Rα and HLA-DR on these cells [49, 65], and also in the functional (i.e. proliferative and cytotoxic) activation of such cells. In fact, PBL of IL-2 treated patients were shown to proliferate and lyse autologous and allogeneic tumours in a TCR-independent and MHC-unrestricted fashion [49], although similar amounts of IL-2 are ten times less effective in vivo than in vitro in inducing LAK activity [66]. Such a loss of activating property by IL-2 in the circulation may have many, disparate explanations such as the presence of soluble IL-2R (which, however, are usually IL-2Rα and not IL-2Rβ), and the release of suppressive factors by the tumour, including TGF-β [14, 67]. The phenotypic and functional properties of immune cells activated by IL-2 are summarised in Table 1.

Table 1. IL-2 activation of different immune cells

Immune cells	Cell surface markers	Cytokine production	Cytotoxicity	Proliferation
T	CD25, DR	yes	small subset	small subset
NK	p55/p70	yes	yes	yes
B	CD25, DR	no	no	small subset
Mø	CD25, DR	yes	yes	no

Cytokine production induced by IL-2

A second, important effect resulting from T and NK activation induced by IL-2 is cytokine production, a phenomenon which can have profound biological and clinical consequences. The cytokines which have been shown to be produced by purified population of T and NK cells or clones upon stimulation with IL-2, as evaluated either at the mRNA or protein level, are summarised in Table 2. T cells stimulated in vitro by IL-2 can produce de novo or increase the basal production of IFN-γ, TNF-α, IL-2, IL-3, IL-4, IL-5, GM-CSF [68-70] whereas NK cells have been described to express IFN-γ, TNF-α and GM-CSF [see 35].

It should be noted, however, that cytokines are expressed in T cells upon stimulation with IL-2 only in the presence of non-antigenic accessory cells and that this pathway of induction is different from that resulting from the TCR-

Table 2. Cytokine expression by T and NK lymphocytes stimulated by IL-2.

Cytokine	T cells	NK cells
IFN-γ	+	+
GM-CSF	+	+
IL-2	+	−
IL-3	+	−
IL-4	+	−
IL-5	+	ND
TNF-α	+	+

ND = not determined

mediated activation [70, 71]. Thus T cells can be activated to release tumour-cytotoxic cytokines both by tumour antigens recognised by the TCR or by IL-2, two processes which may occur either independently or simultaneously at the tumour site resulting in neoplastic cell destruction. The release of tumouricidal cytokines (in particular TNF and/or IFN-γ) induced by IL-2 and anti-TCR/CD3 antibodies may enable non-specific T lymphocytes to overcome intratumour antigenic heterogeneity which limits the effectiveness of MHC-restricted T cells [72]. A possible therapeutic role for cytokines by themselves is suggested by the measurable circulating levels of IFN-γ and TNF-α in IL-2/LAK treated patients [73], and by the correlation between TNF levels and clinical response in such patients [74].

IL-2 is chemotactic for lymphocytes and affects their motility and homing

Another, albeit underscored function of IL-2 is a chemotactic one which serves to recruit lymphocytes at the site of IL-2 production [75]. In addition, IL-2-activated lymphocytes show a greater motility than their unstimulated counterparts although the motile subpopulation, which contains a higher proportion of CD4+ cells, has a lower tumouricidal activity [76] leading the authors to conclude that 'tumour cytotoxicity of circulating lymphocytes may be a misleading indication of the effectiveness of immunotherapy'. Motile subpopulations were subsequently shown to exhibit a twofold greater tumour localization than nonmotile subpopulations in mammary cancer-bearing mice [77]. Thus, these studies suggest that the IL-2-activated lymphocytes contain a fraction with highly motile properties which allow a better targeting to tumour lesions by such lymphocytes which, however, have a low tumouricidal activity. This apparent paradox may in part explain the limited therapeutic activity of LAK cells. Furthermore, IL-2 exposure was shown to decrease the expression of the homing receptor MEL-14 while increasing the adhesion molecule LFA-1 on LAK cells resulting in the lack of localization into lymph nodes in vivo [71]. This reduced localisation of LAK cells into peripheral nodes may explain the low therapeutic activity of LAK and IL-2-based therapy on nodal metastases. In addition, all such changes brought about by IL-2 on the cell surface of activated lymphocytes may explain several effects of the in vivo administration of IL-2 such as the lymphopenia occurring 3-4 hrs after its administration [30] and the accumulation of inflammatory cells at the subcutaneous sites of IL-2 injection [78]. Lymphopenia may also be contributed to by the increased expression of adhesion molecules on endothelial cells induced by the release of cytokines (e.g. IL-1, TNF-α, IFN-γ) by the IL-2-activated lymphocytes and/or macrophages.

Conclusions

IL-2 now has a well defined role, at a molecular level, as a central factor modulating the immune response through its effect on the cells involved in such processes. The discovery that many other cytokines exert a fundamental role in regulating several steps of lymphocyte activation and differentiation by inhibiting or enhancing the activity of IL-2 forces us to reconsider previous conclusions drawn on the basis of the available data. It is important to recognize that T and NK cells, which are the major effectors of a possible antitumour activity, may behave differently when stimulated by IL-2 due to their different expression of IL-2R and production of cytokines. Future immunotherapy studies, therefore, should take into account the knowledge accumulated on mechanisms of action of these two different subsets; such information should translate into a more rational and effective use of cytokines and immune cells in cancer therapy.

Acknowledgements

The author's work was supported by Grants from the Ministry of Public Health (Finalized Oncologic Programs), by the Italy-Usa Program on New Therapy of Tumors (Istituto Superiore Sanità, Rome) and from EuroCetus (Amsterdam).

References

1. Shows T, Eddy R, Haley L, et al. Interleukin 2 (IL2) is assigned to human chromosome 4. Som Cell Mol Genet 1984; 10: 315-20.
2. Wang A, Lu S-D, Mark DF. Site-specific mutagenesis of the human interleukin-2 gene: structure-function analysis of the cysteine residues. Science 1984; 224: 1431-34.
3. Robb RJ, Kutny RM, Panico M, et al. Amino acid sequence and post-translational modifications of human interleukin-2. Proc Natl Acad Sci USA 1984; 81: 8486-91.
4. Taniguchi M, Matsui H, Fujita T, et al. Structure and expression of a cloned cDNA for human interleukin-2. Nature 1983; 302: 305-8.
5. Matsui H, Fujita T, Nishi-Takaoka C, et al. Molecular cloning and expression of the human interleukin-2 gene. In: Pick E, editor. Lymphokine, Vol. 12. New York: Academic Press, 1985: 1-12.
6. Brandhuber BJ, Boone T, Kenney WC, McKay DB. Three-Dimensional Structure of Interleukin-2. Science 1987; 238: 1707-9.

7. Kuo L, Robb RJ. Structure-function relationships for the IL 2-receptor system. J Immunol 1986; 137: 1538-43.
8. Altman A, Cardenas JM, Houghten RA, et al. Antibodies of predetermined specificity against chemically sinthetized peptides of human interleukin 2. Proc Natl Acad Sci USA 1984; 81: 2176-81.
9. Honjo T. Shared patterns in receptors. Curr Opinion Biol 1991; 1: 201-3.
10. Smith KA. Interleukin-2: inception, impact and implications. Science 1988; 240: 1169-76.
11. Phillips JH, Takeshita T, Sugamura K, Lanier LL. Activation of natural killer cells via the p75 interleukin 2 receptor. J Exp Med 1989; 170: 291-6.
12. Saragovi H, Malek T. Proc Natl Acad Sci USA 1990; 87: 11-5.
13. Saito Y, Tada H, Sabe H, Honjo T. Biochemical evidence for a third chain of the interleukin 2 receptor. J Biol Chem 1991; 266: 22186-91.
14. Gambacorti-Passerini C, Rovelli F, Ghezzi R, et al. Serum CD25 levels in patients treated with rIL2 and LAK. Correlation with in vivo immune activation. J Immunol Res 1990; 2: 19-24.
15. Asao H, Takeshita T, Nakamura M, et al. Interleukin 2 (IL-2) induced tyrosine phosphorilation of IL-2 receptor p75. J Exp Med 1990; 171: 637-44.
16. Sharon M, Gnarra JR, Leonard WJ. The β-chain of the IL-2 receptor (p70) is tyrosine-phosphorilated on YT and HUT-102B2 cells. J Immunol 1989; 143, 2530-3.
17. June CH, Fletcher MC, Ledbetter JA, et al. Inhibition of tyrosine phosphorylation prevents T-cell receptor-mediated signal transduction. Proc Natl Acad Sci USA 1990; 87: 7722-26.
18. Horak ID, Gress RE, Lucas PJ, et al. T-lymphocyte interleukin-2 dependent tyrosine protein kinase signal transduction involves the activation of p561ck. Proc Natl Acad Sci USA 1991; 88: 1996-2000.
19. Turner B, Rapp U, Greene M, et al. Interleukin 2 induces tyrosine phosphorilation and activation of p72-74 Raf-1 kinase in a T-cell line. Proc Natl Acad Sci USA 1991; 88: 1227-31.
20. Morrison D, Kaplan D, Escobedo J, et al. Direct activation of the serine/threonine kinase activity of Raf-1 through tyrosine phosphorilation by the PDGF β-receptor. Cell 1989; 58: 649-57.
21. Mond JJ, Thompson C, Finkelman FD, et al. Affinity-purified interleukin 2 induces proliferation of large but not small B cells. Proc Natl Acad Sci USA 1985; 82: 1518-21.
22. Herrmann F, Cannistra SA, Levine H, Griffin JD. Expression of interleukin 2 receptors and binding of interleukin 2 by gamma interferon-induced human leukemic and normal monocyte cells. J Exp Med 1985; 162: 1111-6.
23. Benveniste EN, Merrill JE. Stimulation of oligodendroglial proliferation and maturation by interleukin-2. Nature 1986; 321:610-3.
24. Steiner G, Tschachler E, Tani M, et al. Interleukin-2 receptors on cultured murine epidermal Langherans cells. J Immunol 1986; 137: 155-9.
25. Benveniste EN, Herman PK, Whitaker JN. Myelin basic protein-specific RNA levels in interleukin-2-stimulated oligodendrocytes. J Neurochem 1987; 49: 1274-9.
26. Plaisance S, Rubinstein E, Alileche A, et al. Human melanoma cells express an IL-2R, which is involved in the modulation of the ICAM-1 protein. Proc. Am Ass Cancer Res 1991; 31: 240.
27. Malkovska V, Murphy J, Hudson L, Bevan D. Direct effect of interleukin-2 on chronic lymphocytic leukemia B cell function and morphology. Clin Exp Immunol 1987; 68: 677-84.
28. Yamamoto S, Hattori T, Matsuoka M, et al. Induction of Tac antigen and proliferation of myeloid leukemic cells by ATL-derived factor: comparison with other agents that promote differentiation of human myeloid or monocytic leukemic cells. Blood 1986; 67: 1713-20.
29. Estrov Z, Freedman MH. Growth requirements for human acute lymphoblastic leukemia cells: refinement of a clonogenic assay. Cancer Res 1988; 48: 2372-6.
30. Lotze MT, Matory YL, Ettinghausen SE, et al. In vivo administration of purified human interleukin 2. II. Half-life, immunologic effects, and expansion of peripheral lymphoid cells in vivo with recombinant interleukin-2. J Immunol 1985; 135: 2865-75.
31. Meuer SC, Hussey R, Cantrell DA, et al. Triggering of the T3-Ti antigen-receptor complex results in clonal T-cell proliferation through an interleukin 2-dependent autocrine pathway.

Proc Natl Acad Sci USA 1984; 81: 1509-13.
32. Dianzani U, Zarcone D, Pistoia V, et al. CD8+/CD11b+ peripheral blood T lymphocytes contain lymphokine-activated killer cell precursors. Eur J Immunol 1989; 19: 1037-44.
33. Silvennoinen O, Vakkila J, Hurme M. Accessory cells, dendritic cells, or monocytes are required for the lymphokine-activated killer cell induction from resting T cells but not from natural killer cell precursors. J Immunol 1988; 141: 1404-9.
34. Lenardo MJ. Interleukin-2 programs mouse $\alpha\beta$ T lymphocytes for apoptosis. Nature 1991; 353: 858-61.
35. Perussia B. Lymphokine-activated killer cells, natural killer cells and cytokines. Curr Opin Immunol 1991; 3: 49-55.
36. London P, Perussia B, Trinchieri G. Induction of proliferation in vitro of resting human natural killer cells: IL-2 induces into cell cycle most peripheral blood NK cells, but only a minor subset of low density T cells. J Immunol 1986; 137: 3845-54.
37. Tsudo M, Goldman CK, Bongiovanni KF, et al. The p75 peptide is the receptor for interleukin-2 expressed on a large granular lymphocytes and is responsible for the interleukin-2 activation of these cells. Proc Natl Acad Sci USA 1987; 84: 5394-8.
38. Kobayashi M, Fitz L, Ryan M, et al. Identification and purification of natural killer cell stimulatory factor (NKSF). J Exp Med 1989; 170: 827-46.
39. Smyth MJ, Ortaldo JR. Comparison of the effect of IL-2 and IL-6 on the lytic activity of purified human peripheral blood large granular lymphocytes. J Immunol 1991; 146: 1380-4.
40. Naume B, Espevik T. Effects of IL-7 and IL-2 on highly enriched CD56+ natural killer cells. A comparative study. J Immunol 1991; 147: 2208-14.
41. Vaage JT, Reynolds CW, Reynolds D, et al. The proliferation and life-span of rat large granular lymphocytes: effects of cytokines. Eur J Immunol 1989; 19: 1895-1902.
42. Spits H, Yssel H, Pallard X, et al. IL-4 inhibits IL-2 mediated induction of human lymphokine-activated killer cells, but not the generation of antigen-specific cytotoxic T lymphocytes in mixed leukocyte cultures. J Immunol 1988; 141: 29-36.
43. Owen-Schaub LB, Crump WL III, Morin GI, Grimm EA. Regulation of lymphocyte tumor-necrosis factor receptors by IL-2. J Immunol 1989; 143: 2236-41.
44. Naume B, Shalaby R, Lesslauer W, Espevik T. Involvement of the 55- and 75-KDa tumor necrosis factor receptors in the generation of lymphokine-activated killer cell activity and proliferation of natural killer cells. J Immunol 1991; 146: 3045-8.
45. Chen W, Reese VA, Cheever MA. Adoptively transferred antigen-specific T cells can be grown and maintained in large numbers in vivo for extended periods of time by intermittent restimulation with specific antigen plus IL-2. J Immunol 1990; 144: 3659-66.
46. Rodolfo M, Bassi C, Salvi C, Parmiani G. Therapeutic use of a long-term cytotoxic T cell line recognizing a common tumour-associated antigen: the pattern of in vitro reactivity predicts the in vivo effect on different tumours. Cancer Immunol Immunother 1991; 34: 53-62.
47. Biron CA, Young HA, Kasauani NT. Interleukin-2-induced proliferation of murine natural killer cells in vivo. J Exp Med 1990; 171: 173-88.
48. Ellis TM, Creekmore SP, McMannis JD, et al. Appearance and phenotypic characterization of circulating Leu19+ cells in cancer patients receiving recombinant interleukin 2. Cancer Res 1988; 48: 6597-6602.
49. Gambacorti-Passerini C, Radrizzani M, Marolda R, et al. In vivo activation of lymphocytes in melanoma patients receiving escalating doses of recombinant interleukin 2. Int J Cancer 1988; 41: 700-6.
50. Schorle H, Holtschke T, Hunig T, et al. Development and function of T cells in mice rendered interleukin-2 deficient by gene targeting. Nature 1991; 352: 621-4.
51. Swain SL. Lymphokine and the immune response: the central role of interleukin-2. Curr Opin Immunol 1991; 3: 304-10.
52. Kishimoto T. The biology of interleukin-6. Blood 1989; 74: 1-10.
53. Okazaki H, Ito M, Sudo T, et al. IL-7 promotes thymocyte proliferation and maintains immunocompetent thymocytes bearing $\alpha\beta$ or $\gamma\delta$ T-cell receptors in vitro: synergism with IL-2.

J Immunol 1989; 143: 2917-22.
54. Malkovsky M, Lovelan B, North M, et al. Recombinant interleukin-2 directly augments the cytotoxicity of human monocytes. Nature 1987; 325: 262-5.
55. Tentori L, Longo DL, Zuniga-Pflucker JC, et al. Essential role of the interleukin-2-receptor pathway in thymocyte maturation in vivo. J Exp Med 1988; 168: 1741-8.
56. Leist TP, Kohler M, Eppler M, Zinkernagel RM. Effects of treatment with IL-2 receptor specific monoclonal antibody in mice: inhibition of cytotoxic T cell responses but not by T helper. J Immunol 1989; 143: 628-32.
57. Parmiani G, Anichini A, Fossati G. Cellular imune response against autologous human malignant melanoma: are in vistro studies providing a framework for a more effective immunotherapy? J Natl Cancer Inst 1990; 82: 361-70.
58. Smyth MJ, Ortaldo JR, Bere W, et al. IL-2 and IL-6 synergize to augment the performing protein gene expression and cytotoxic potential of human peripheral blood T cells. J Immunol 1990: 145: 1159-66.
59. Chen W-F, Zlotnik A. IL-10: a novel cytotoxic T cell differentiation factor. J Immunol 1991; 147: 528-34.
60. Roder J. Killing comes naturally. Curr Biol 1991; 1: 242-4.
61. Xiao J, Brahmi Z. Target cell-directed inactivation and IL-2 dependent reactivation of LAK cells. Cell Immunol 1989; 122: 295-306.
62. Sone S, Utsugi T, Nii A, Ogura T. Differential effects of recombinant interferons α, β and γ on induction of human lymphokine (IL-2)-activated killer activity. J Natl Cancer Inst 1988; 80: 425-31.
63. Grimm EA, Mazumder A, Zhang HZ, et al. Lymphokine-activated killer cell phenomenon. Lysis of natural killer-resistant fresh solid tumor cells by interleukin-2-activated autologous human peripheral blood lymphocyte. J Exp Med 1982; 155: 1823-41.
64. Phillips JH, Lanier LL. Dissection of the lymphokine-activated killer phenomenon. Relative contribution of peripheral blood natural killer cells and T lymphocytes to cytolysis. J Exp Med 1986; 164: 814-25.
65. Lotze M, Custer MC, Sharrow SO, et al. In vivo administration of purified human interleukin-2 to patients with cancer: development of interleukin-2 receptor following interleukin-2 administration. Cancer Res. 1987; 47: 2188-95.
66. Gambacorti-Passerini C, Rivoltini L, Radrizzani M, et al. Differences between in vivo and in vitro activation of cancer patient lymphocytes by recombinant interleukin-2: possible role for lymphokine-activated killer cell infusion in the in vivo-induced activation. Cancer Res 1989; 49: 5230-4.
67. Grimm EA, Crump WL III, Durett A, et al. TGF-β inhibits the in vitro induction of lymphokine-activated killing activity. Cancer Immunol Immunother 1988; 27; 27: 53-8.
68. Farrar WJ, Johnson HM, Farrar JJ, Regulation of the production of immune interferon and cytotoxic T lymphocytes by interleukin-2. J Immunol 1981; 126: 1120-5.
69. Dunn DE, Jin J, Lancki DW, Fitch FW. An alternate pathway of induction of lymphokine production by T lymphocyte clones. J Immunol 1989; 142: 3847-56.
70. Enokihara H, Furusawa S, Nakakubo H, et al. T cell from eosinophilic patients produce interleukin-2 with interleukin-5 stimulation. Blood 1989; 73: 1809-13.
71. Steen PD, McGregor JR, Lehman CM, Samlowski WE. Changes in homing receptor expression on murine lymphokine activated killer cells during IL-2 exposure. J Immunol 1989; 143: 4324-30.
72. Mazzocchi A, Rodolfo M, Parmiani G, Anichini A. An autologous T cell clone overcomes intra-melanoma heterogeneity for susceptibility to cell-mediated lysis by using multiple lytic mechanisms: in vitro and in vivo analysis. Melanoma Res 1991; 1: 169-76.
73. Gemlo BT, Palladino MA, Jaffe HS, et al. Circulating cytokines in patients with metastatic cancer treated with recombinant interleukin-2 and lymphokine-activated killer cells. Cancer Res 1988; 48: 5864-7.
74. Blay J-Y, Favrot MC, Negrier S, et al. Correlation between clinical response to interleukin-2

therapy and sustained production of tumor necrosis factor. Cancer Res 1990; 50: 2371-4.
75. Kornfeld H, Berman JS, Beer DJ, Center DM. Induction of human T lymphocyte motility by interleukin-2. J Immunol 1985; 134: 3887-90.
76. Ratner S, Heppner GH. Motility and tumoricidal activity of interleukin-2-stimulated lymphocytes. Cancer Res 1988; 48: 3374-80.
77. Ratner S. Lymphocytes stimulated with recombinant human interleukin-2: relationship between motility into protein matrix and in vivo localization in normal and neoplastic tissues of mice. J Natl Cancer Inst 1990; 82: 612-16.
78. Whitehead RP, Ward D, Hemingway L, et al. Subcutaneous recombinant interleukin-2 in a dose escalating regimen in patients with metastatic renal cell adenocarcinoma. Cancer Res 1990; 50: 6708-15.

6. Interleukin-2 and tumour eradication by cytotoxic T lymphocytes

CORNELIS J.M. MELIEF and W. MARTIN KAST

Introduction

So far the most effective arm of the immune response against both virus- and non-virus-induced tumours is T-cell immunity (reviewed in [1–4]). The principles of T-cell immunity against virus-induced tumours are the same as those against viruses in general. Small immunogenic peptides, processed from viral proteins are presented, bound to MHC class I or class II molecules at the surface of tumour cells or associated antigen presenting cells to CD8 cytotoxic T (T_C) cells or CD4+ T helper (T_H) cells, respectively. Recent studies indicate that non-virus-induced tumours of experimental animals and human beings can also evoke T-cell responses against non-mutated gene products. These responses [5, 6] may have similar protective or therapeutic potential as the T cell responses against virus-induced tumours.

Tumour infiltrating lymphocytes (TIL) consist of mixed populations of cells including CD4+ and CD8+ T lymphocytes that may or may not be tumour specific and natural killer (NK) cells. Obviously, the coexistence in patients of tumour masses infiltrated with lymphocytes shows that the tumour eradicating potential of these cells is not sufficient. IL-2 is a most powerful cytokine with the capacity to tip the balance from coexistence of cancer and TIL towards complete tumour eradication by TIL. So far this capacity of IL-2 has not yet been exploited to the full extent, mainly because isolation of the most active tumour specific T lymphocytes from TIL has not been accomplished. Also, identification of the molecular target structures of tumour specific T-cells is only in its infancy. If eventually the molecular target structures of tumour specific T-cells are known, therapy with adoptively transferred TIL and IL-2 can be combined with or even replaced by tumour specific peptide vaccination with or without additional IL-2.

J. Wagstaff (ed.), The Role of Interleukin-2 in the Treatment of Cancer Patients, 85-94.

Mechanism of antigen recognition by T-cells

T-cells recognise small peptides bound to the antigen presenting groove of MHC class I molecules (CD8+ Tc cells) or MHC class II molecules (CD4+ T_H cells). The CD8+ Tc cells have the most powerful anti-tumour activity, although tumour eradication by non-cytotoxic CD4+ T_H clones has also been reported [1–4], even against MHC class II negative tumours. The expression of MHC class II antigens is largely restricted to cells of the lymphohemopoietic lineage and tumours originating thereof.

Abnormal MHC class II expression is found on certain tumours such as human melanoma. Expression of MHC class I antigens occurs in most nucleated cells and derived tumours, but vast differences in expression are found. Down-regulation of MHC class I expression is one of the devious tricks by which tumour cells evade immune attack by CD8+ Tc (reviewed in [3, 7]).

The processing pathways for presentation of peptides by MHC class I molecules differ from those involved in presentation of peptides by MHC class II molecules. MHC class I molecules are loaded in the endoplasmic reticulum (ER) with peptides pumped from the cytosol by molecules functioning as peptide pumps, at least some of which are encoded by the MHC [8–11]. The peptides themselves are generated by so-called proteasomes in the cytosol, likewise encoded by the MHC, that generate peptide fragments from proteins [12, 13]. Peptides for presentation by MHC class II molecules, on the other hand, do not enter the MHC class II molecule in the ER, because access to the MHC class II antigen presenting groove is selectively blocked by the invariant (li) chain [14, 15]. The same li chain appears to direct traffic of MHC class II molecules towards the endosomal lysosomal pathway [16]. Due to low pH conditions in the late endosomes/lysosomes and proteolytic activity, the li chain detaches from the antigen presenting groove and MHC class II molecules can be loaded with immunogenic fragments generated in the endosomal/lysosomal compartment from proteins derived from e.g. the cell surface or endocytosed from the exterior of the cell. Thus in general the MHC class I pathway is specialised in the presentation of cytosol derived peptides while MHC class II is specialised in the presentation of exogenous and cell surface derived material.

The enormous variability in T cell receptors capable of recognising a universe of different MHC peptide complexes arises by genetic recombination between T cell receptor variable and constant region genes in a manner very similar to that of the generation of diversity in immunoglobulin molecules. The most common T-cell receptor is the $\alpha\beta$ T-cell receptor, consisting of an α, β heterodimer. Each α and β chain is composed of variable and constant region gene products.

Size of peptides recognised by cytotoxic and helper T lymphocytes

For immunogenic peptides binding to MHC class I molecules a fairly rigorous length requirement exists of 8–11 amino acids, due to the fact that these peptides fit snugly into the MHC class I groove, that appears to be closed at both ends of the groove [17–20]. Peptides optimally binding to the groove of MHC class II molecules are probably larger (12–16 amino acids) than those binding to MHC class I, perhaps because the peptide binding groove of MHC class II molecules may be open at either or both extremities [21].

MHC allele specific motifs in MHC class I binding peptides

Viral peptides involved in T_C recognition as well as self peptides eluted from MHC class I molecules have recently been found to contain allele specific amino acid motifs. These motifs are characterised by the presence of one or two dominant 'anchor' residues at fixed allele specific positions in the peptide (e.g. L or M at position 2 and V at position 9, of HLA-A2.1 binding peptides [20] and arginine at position 2 in HLA-B27 [22]). These 'anchor' residues are involved in binding to allele specific pockets in the MHC class I antigen presenting groove [22].

In addition, 'strong' and 'weak' residues at other positions in the peptide can be distinguished, i.e. residues that occur high or less high above background in material eluted from the groove of specific MHC class I molecules [20].

These peptide profiles allow prediction of sequences in proteins that are likely to be processed and to bind to individual MHC class I alleles. Known T_C epitopes of viruses, bacteria, parasites and tumour antigens generally follow these rules [20, 23], although exceptions may occur. These allele specific motifs allow prediction of potential T_C epitopes in target molecules of choice in tumours [4].

Tumour eradication by adoptive transfer of T lymphocytes and IL-2 in animal models

Murine Leukemia Virus in Mice (MuLV) specific T_C directed against both envelope (env) and internal (gag) gene products of both AKV/Gross and Friend/Moloney/Rauscher viruses have been reported in mice [24–26]. In the case of Friend virus induced leukemias of H-2^b mice, I-A^b restricted T_H clones were directed against an env product whereas H-$2D^b$ restricted T_C were directed against a gag product [25]. T_H and T_C clones were capable of eradicating disseminated FBL3 Friend leukaemia [1] upon adoptive transfer in tumour bearing animals, illustrating the tumour rejection potential of both the T_H and T_C subsets of T cells.

In this model some FBL3 specific T_C clones produce sufficient IL-2 to exert a marked therapeutic effect without a requirement for exogenous IL-2 [1, 3]. However, addition of high dose exogenous IL-2 further enhances the therapeutic efficacy of these adoptively transferred T_C.

Eradication of MHC class I negative FBL3 Friend leukemia cells by MHC class II restricted CD4 clones is remarkable and is probably brought about by the induction of tumoricidal activity in macrophages, induced by Interferon-*y*, secreted by the CD4+ FBL3 specific T cells [1]. In this model successful adoptive therapy requires combined treatment with cyclophosfamide.

In a human Adenovirus induced tumour model developed in our laboratory large tumour masses in T cell deficient nude mice can be eradicated by adoptive transfer of approximately 15×10^6 tumour specific CD8+ cloned Tc, directed against the nuclear oncogene encoded peptide SGPSNTPPEI [27]. No additional chemotherapy or irradiation is required in this model. Because these T_C are entirely IL-2 dependent, effective therapy requires simultaneous administration of recombinant IL-2 (10^5 units in incomplete Freund adjuvant, allowing slow delivery of IL-2). This 10-mer peptide is presented by the H-2D^b MHC class I molecule [27, 28]. Binding of the peptide to H-2D^b can be easily demonstrated by stabilisation of empty H-2 D^b molecules at the surface of antigen processing defective RMA-S cells [28].

Adoptive transfer studies with bulk populations and clones of tumour-specific T cells have been very useful in demonstrating the power of T cell immunity in tumour eradication [1–4]. On the other hand for clinical purposes adoptive transfer is labour intensive, cumbersome and costly and is therefore unlikely to allow widespread clinical applications as an efficient form of immunotherapy of cancer. Indeed, although some beneficial effects were attributed to therapy with IL-2 and lymphokine activated killer cells or expanded tumour infiltrating lymphocytes in comparison to treatment with IL-2 alone in patients with melanoma and renal cell carcinoma [3], logistic problems have so far prevented cancer therapy with cloned tumour-specific T cells. This leads one to ponder alternatives that may circumvent these difficulties. A promising possibility to explore is vaccination with immunodominant peptides (see below).

Tumour specific cytotoxic T cells in human cancer and therapy with adoptive transfer of such cells

Class I MHC restricted tumour specific T_C have been cultured from peripheral blood lymphocytes or from TIL in patients with melanoma, kidney carcinoma or carcinoma of the ovary [3, 29]. No therapeutic attempts have been made with cloned tumour specific CTL, but trials with IL-2 expanded populations of TIL's have shown beneficial effects in patients with melanoma and renal cell carcinoma, although the duration of remissions was usually short [30–32]. These bulk populations of TIL contained varying numbers of CD4+ and CD8+ cells. Either population may have contained tumour specific T-cells, notably CD8+ T_C as the most active therapeutic principle. Further proof of this contention must come from therapy with cloned tumour specific T cells in combination with IL-2.

Peptide vaccination for generation of protective Tc

Recent studies indicate that vaccination with immunodominant peptides may be very effective in protection against viruses and virus-induced tumours. Subcutaneous vaccination with immunodominant peptides presented by MHC class I molecules using incomplete Freund adjuvant (FA) as a slow release vehicle, was effective in inducing a strong memory T_C response associated with reduced titers of lymphocytochoriomeningitis virus (LCMV) [33] or protection against Sendai virus pneumonia [24]. In a third study priming of influenza virus-specific T_C in vivo was achieved by peptide vaccination [34], but in this case the peptide-immune mice were not significantly protected from viral infection [35]. The first indication that peptide vaccination can protect against tumours was obtained in a polyoma virus model in mice [36]. The prevalence in these peptides of T_H and T_C epitopes was not analysed, however.

In our studies on protection against Sendai pneumonia, peptide length requirements for optimal vaccine protection were much less rigorous than in H-2 binding assays. In our original publication a 16 mer of the Sendai nucleoprotein was used for vaccination [34]. Later studies [49] have shown that the amount of 16 mer required for optimal induction of T_C mediated protection is the same as that of the optimally binding 9 mer FAPGNYPAL [19]. Presumably the 16 mer is efficiently broken down in vivo to the 9 mer, perhaps by Langerhans cells in the skin.

An intriguing question in vaccination with MHC class I binding peptides is, to which extent simultaneous activation in vivo of CD4+ T cells is required. In studies with the LCMV peptide it was found that this peptide also contains a T_H epitope that stimulates CD4+ cells. The simultaneous stimulation by both the T_H and T_C epitopes in this peptide was deemed necessary for optimal T_C memory induction [37]. On the other hand, there is no evidence that vaccination with the immunodominant Sendai virus peptide studied in our laboratory in H-2^b mice requires simultaneous activation of CD4+ cells. This peptide sequence does not contain a T_H epitope (W.M. Kast and C.J.M. Melief, unpublished observations). Possibly the particular characteristics of the T_C epitope, such as affinity of binding to MHC class I molecules, determine the need for simultaneous CD4+ T-cell activation during priming. In our hands both the Sendai virus NP and Adeno virus E1A immumodominant T_C peptides can generate T_C responses in T-cells from unprimed mice in vitro in the absence of CD4+ T-cells if presented on processing defective RMA-S cells [38] or dendritic cells [39]. Earlier studies have also suggested that CD8+ T_C responses induced by dendritic cells are entirely CD4+ T_H cell independent [40, 41].

Target molecules for tumour specific T-lymphocytes in human cancer

In a previous review we have proposed a novel strategy for generation of tumour specific T-cells [4]. This strategy does not depend on expansion of tumour infiltrating lymphocytes but rather intentionally directs T-cells to respond to target molecules of choice in the neoplastic cells. Such antigens can be viral antigens in virus-induced tumour cells. In non-virus induced tumour cells, desirable target molecules are differentiation antigens of restricted tissue distribution, overexpressed or mutated oncogene products including point mutations and chromosomal breakpoint peptides. The list of target molecules against which we and others have generated T_C or are trying to generate T_C is shown in Table 1

Table 1. Target molecules of choice for cytotoxic T lymphocytes directed against human cancer

Tumour type	Virus	Target molecule
I. Virus-induced tumours		
- Cervical carcinoma	Human papilloma virus types 16 & 18 (HPV16 & 18)	Early region 6 and early region 7 of HPV16 and HPV18
- Burkitt's lymphoma	Epstein-Barr virus (EBV)	EBNA 1?
- Adult T-cell leukemia lymphoma	Human T lymphotropic virus I	?
II. Non-virus induced tumours		
- Many different malignancies		Mutated or overexpressed p53
- Sarcomas		Overexpressed mdm2
- Various malignancies		Mutated ras
- Chronic myelogenous leukemia		bcr/abl breakpoint peptide
- Melanoma		Melanoma associated gene products (MAGE)
- B lymphoma		CD19 & CD20 B lymphocyte differentiation antigens Immunoglobulin idiotypes

In a number of instances T_C against the target structures listed in Table 1 were found naturally in PBL from cancer patients or in the case of EBV, healthy EBV carriers. By elegant gene cloning technology a melanoma associated gene (MAGE) family was identified using HLA-A1 presented MAGE peptide recognition by T_C as a gene product recognition system [6].

With the help of vaccinia virus recombinants individually expressing each of the eight EBV latent proteins normally found in lymphoblastoid cell lines, EBNA 3A, 3B and 3C were identified as frequent T_C target structures in donors with a variety of MHC types [42]. The precise peptides recognised are not yet known, nor is it known whether these T_C have anti-tumour activity against EBV associated malignancies. Various groups have successfully generated specific T cells against mutated ras peptides [43], including ourselves (unpublished observations).

Cervical cancer is strongly associated with human papilloma virus (HPV) infection, notably HPV16 and HPV18 [44]. The transforming regions E6 and E7 of HPV16 and HPV18 interact with the cellular p53 and retinoblastoma (Rb) tumour suppressor gene products, respectively. These interactions are probably important steps in the sequence of events towards malignancy [44]. In non-virus-induced tumours p53 is frequently deleted or mutated, in the latter case associated with overexpression of p53 [45]. Recently it was found that in a high proportion of sarcomas the growth suppressing function of p53 is inactivated by binding of the MDM-2 oncogene product to the p53 protein [46–48]. In human sarcomas the MDM-2 gene was found to be amplified to exert this function [47]. Overexpressed MDM-2, like overexpressed p53, is a potential target for tumour specific Tc.

Recently we have embarked on the generation of Tc against HPV16 and p53 using the following strategy: overlapping peptides or 'motif' bearing peptides were screened for binding to the appropriate MHC class I molecules. After establishment of binding, these peptides were used either to immunise mice or to induce primary in vitro T_C responses both in mice and humans. In the case of HPV16 induced tumours in mice one of the identified peptides was indeed able to induce protective immunity against HPV16 induced tumours (M.C.W. Feltkamp, C.J.M. Melief and W.M. Kast, unpublished observations). Since this effect was already achieved without apparent help by IL-2 producing CD4+ cells, because only a T_C epitope was used, it will be worthwhile to test if addition of IL-2 would improve the effect of the immunisation. In the case of p53, binding peptides were identified that bind to the human HLA-A2.1 allele. It was possible to induce human primary T_C responses and even T_C clones against these peptides (J. Houbiers, H.W. Nijman, W.M. Kast and C.J.M. Melief, unpublished observations). These T_C clones will be tested on tumour cells with overexpressed p53 that bear the appropriate HLA-A2.1 molecule. The MHC restricted nature of T_C recognition of course causes the problem that many different peptides of the same protein have to be identified for the many different HLA alleles. However, if one would aim for the most frequent ones such as HLA-A1, A2 and A3, already 90 per cent of the Caucasian population would be covered, indicating that not many different peptides would have to be identified.

Epilogue

Immunotherapy of tumours by adoptive transfer of cytotoxic T cells T_C is now feasible in experimental murine systems. These T_C recognise peptide sequences of defined length presented in the groove of MHC class I molecules. Effective eradication of large tumour masses requires co-administration of IL-2. Tumour escape strategies are numerous, but in various instances can be counteracted by defined measures. Initiation of T_C responses against poorly immunogenic non-virus-induced tumours (the majority of human cancer) requires novel strategies to overcome T cell inertia. Rather than wait-and-see whether tumour specific T_C (against unknown antigens) can be cultured from tumour infiltrating lymphocytes we propose an alternative strategy in which T_C are raised against target molecules of choice including differentiation antigens of restricted tissue distribution (autoantigens) or mutated/overexpressed oncogene products. The various steps proposed include:

1. Identification of target molecules of choice.
2. Identification in these target molecules of MHC allele specific peptide motifs involved in peptide binding to MHC molecules.
3. Evaluation of actual binding of such peptides to specific MHC class I molecules.
4. In vitro T_C response induction by such peptides, presented by highly efficient antigen presenting cells such as processing defective cells, carrying empty MHC class I molecules, loaded with a single peptide or dendritic cells. Both types of cells are capable of primary T_C response induction in vitro.
5. Adoptive transfer of tumour specific T_C generated in vitro or, more convenient, vaccination with immunodominant peptides.

These various steps have now been taken for several viruses, viral induced tumours and other types of tumours and the first indications that this strategy is useful have been obtained.

Acknowledgements

Our work reported in this review was supported by the Dutch Cancer Society and by the Netherlands Organisation for Scientific Research. W.M. Kast is a fellow of the Royal Netherlands Academy of Arts and Sciences.

References

1. Greenberg PD, Klarnet JP, Kern DE, Cheever MA. Therapy of disseminated tumours by adoptive transfer of specifically immune T cells. Prog Exp Tumour Res 1988; 32: 104–27.
2. North RJ, Awwad M, Dunn PC. T cell mediated tumour regression in experimental systems. In: F Melchers, editor. Progression Immunology. 1989; 7: 1097–163.
3. Melief CJM. Tumour eradication by adoptive transfer of cytotoxic T lymphocytes. Adv Cancer Res 1992; 58: 143–75.
4. Melief CJM, Kast WM. Lessons from T cell responses to virus induced tumours for cancer eradication in general. Cancer Surv 1992; 13: 81–99.
5. Van den Eynde B, Lethé B, van Pel A, et al. The gene coding for a major tumour rejection antigen of tumour p815 is identical to the normal gene of syngeneic DBA/2 mice. J Exp Med

1991; 173: 1373–84.
6. Van der Bruggen P, Traversari C, Chomez P, et al. A gene encoding an antigen recognized by cytotoxic T lymphocytes on a human melanoma. Science 1991; 254: 1643–7.
7. Melief CJM, Kast WM. Cytotoxic T lymphocyte therapy of cancer and tumour escape mechanisms. Seminars in Cancer Biology 1991; Vol. II: 347–54.
8. Deverson EV, Gow IR, Coadwell WJ, et al. MHC Class II region encoding proteins related to the multidrug resistance family of transmembrane transporters. Nature 1990; 348: 738–41.
9. Trowsdale J, Hanson I, Mockridge I, et al. Sequences encoded in the class II region of the MHC related to the 'ABC' superfamily of transporters. Nature 1990; 348: 738–41.
10. Spies T, Breslauer M, Bahrain S, et al. A gene in the human major histocompatibility class II region controlling the class I presentation pathway. Nature 1990; 348: 744–7.
11. Monaco JJ, Cho S, Attaya M. Transport protein genes in the murine MHC: possible implications for antigen processing. Science 1990; 250: 1723–6.
12. Brown MG, Driscoll J, Monaco JJ. Structural and serological similarity of MHC-linked LMP and proteasome (multicatalytic proteinase) complexes. Nature 1991; 353: 355–7.
13. Glynne R, Powis SH, Beck S, et al. A proteasome-related gene between the two ABC transporter loci in the class II region of the human MHC. Nature 1991; 353: 357–60.
14. Roche PA, Cresswell P. Invariant chain association with HLA DR molecules inhibits immunogeneic peptide binding. Nature 1990; 345: 615–7.
15. Teyton L, O'Sullivan D, Dickson PW, et al. Invariant chain distinguishes between the exogeneous and endogeneous antigen presentation pathways. Nature 1990; 348: 39–44.
16. Bakke O, Dobberstein B. MHC Class II associated invariant chain contains a sorting signal for endosomal compartments. Cell 1990; 63: 707–16.
17. Van Bleek G, Nathenson SG. Isolation of an endogeneously processed immunodominant viral peptide from the class I H-2 K^b molecule. Nature 1990; 348: 213–6.
18. Rötschke O, Falk F, Deres K, et al. Isolation and analysis of naturally processed viral peptides as recognized by cytotoxic T cells. Nature 1990; 348: 252–4.
19. Schumacher TNM, de Bruijn MLH, Vernie LN, et al. Peptide selection by MHC class I molecules. Nature 1991; 350: 703–6.
20. Falk K, Rötschke O, Stevanovic S, et al. Allele specific motifs revealed by sequencing of self-peptides eluted from MHC molecules. Nature 1991; 351: 290–6.
21. Rudensky AY, Preston-Hurlburt P, Hong SC, et al. Sequence analysis of peptides bound to MHC class II molecules. Nature 1991; 353: 622–7.
22. Madden DR, Gorga JC, Strominger JL, Wiley DC. The structure of HLA-B27 reveals nonamer self-peptides bound in an extended conformation. Nature 1991; 353: 321–5.
23. Pamer EG, Harly JT, Bevan MJ. Precise prediction of a dominant class I MHC-restricted epitope of Listeria monocytogenes. Nature 1991; 353: 852–5.
24. Plata F, Langlade-Demoyen P, Abastado JP, et al. Retrovirus antigens recognized by cytotoxic T lymphocytes activate tumour rejection in vivo. Cell 1987; 48: 231–40.
25. Klarnet JP, Kern DE, Okuno K, et al. FBL-reactive CD8+ cytotoxic and CD4+ helper T lymphocytes recognize distinct Friend murine leukemic virus-encoded antigens. J Exp Med 1989; 169: 457–67.
26. Ke-San Ruan, Lilly F. Identification of an epitope encoded in the env gene of Friend murine leukemia virus, recognized by anti-Friend virus cytotoxic T lymphocytes. Virology 1991; 181: 91–100.
27. Kast WM, Offringa R, Peters PJ, et al. Eradication of Adenovirus E1 induced tumours by E1A specific cytotoxic T lymphocytes. Cell 1989; 59: 603–14.
28. Kast WM, Melief CJM. Fine specificity of cytotoxic T lymphocytes directed against Adenovirus-induced tumours and peptide-MHC binding. Int J Cancer 1991(Suppl)6: 90–4.
29. Ioannides CG, Platsoncas CD, Rasked S, et al. Tumour cytolosis by lymphocytes infiltrating ovarian malignant ascites. Cancer Res 1991; 51: 4257–65.
30. Rosenberg SA, Packard BS, Aebersold PM, et al. Use of tumour infiltrating lymphocytes and interleukin-2 in the immunotherapy of patients with metastatic melanoma: a preliminary

report. New Engl J Med 1988; 319: 1676–80.
31. Fisher B, Packard BS, Read EJ, et al. Tumour localisation of adoptively transferred indium-111 labeled tumour infiltrating lymphocytes in patients with metastatic melanoma. J Clin Oncol 1989; 7: 250–61.
32. Kradin RL, Kurnick JT, Lazarus DS, et al. Tumour infiltrating lymphocytes and interleukin-2 in treatment of advanced cancer. Lancet 1989; 1: 577–80.
33. Schulz M, Zinkernagel RH, Hengartner H. Peptide-induced antiviral protection by cytotoxic T cells. Proc Natl Acad Sci USA 1991; 88: 991-3.
34. Kast WM, Roux L, Curran J, et al. Protection against lethal Sendai virus infection by in vivo priming of virus-specific cytotoxic T lymphocytes with a free synthetic peptide. Proc Natl Acad Sci USA 1991; 88: 2283–7.
35. Gao X-M, Zheng B, Liew FY, et al. Priming of influenza virus-specific cytotoxic T lymphocytes in vivo by short synthetic peptides. J Immunol 1991; 147: 3268–73.
36. Reinkoldsson-Ljunggren G, Ramqvist T, Ärklund-Richter L, Dalianis T. Immunization against polyoma tumours with synthetic peptides derived from the sequences of middle - and large - T antigens. Int J Cancer 1992; 50: 142–6.
37. Fayolle C, Deriand E, Leclerc C. In vivo induction of cytotoxic T cell response by a free synthetic peptide requires CD4+ T cell help. J Immunol 1991; 147: 4069–73.
38. De Bruijn MHL, Schumacher TNM, Nieland JD, et al. Peptide loading of empty major histocompatibility complex molecules on RMA-S cells allows induction of primary cytotoxic T lymphocyte responses. Eur J Immunol 1991; 21: 2963–70.
39. De Bruijn MLH, Nieland JD, Schumacher TNM, et al. Mechanisms of induction of primary virus-specific cytotoxic T lymphocyte responses. Eur J Immunol. In Press.
40. Inaba K, Young JW, Steinman ERM. Direct activation of CD8+ cytotoxic T lymphocytes by dendritic cells. J Exp Med 1987; 166: 182–94.
41. Boog CJP, Boes J, Melief CJM. Stimulation with dendritic cells decreases or obviates the CD4+ helper cell requirement in cytotoxic T lymphocyte responses. Eur J Immunol 1988; 18: 219–23.
42. Murray RJ, Kurilla MG, Brooks JM, et al. Identification of target antigens for the human cytotoxic T lymphocyte response to Epstein-Barr virus (EBV): implications for the immune control of EBV-positive malignancies. J Exp Med 1992; 176: 157–68.
43. Jung S, Schluesener HJ. Human T lymphocytes recognize a peptide of single point-mutated oncogenic ras proteins. J Exp Med 1991; 173: 273–6.
44. Zur Hausen H. Viruses in human cancers. Science 1991; 243: 1167–73.
45. Weinberg RA. Tumor suppressor genes. Science 1991; 243: 1138–46.
46. Momand J, Zambetti GP, Olson DC, et al. The mdm-2 oncogene product forms a complex with the p53 protein and inhibits p53-mediated transactivation. Cell 1992; 69: 1237–45.
47. Oliner JD, Kinzler KW, Meltzer PS, et al. Amplification of a gene encoding a p53-associated protein in human sarcomas. Nature 1992; 358: 80–3.
48. Lane DP. p53, guardian of the genome. Nature 1992; 358: 15–6.
49. Kast WM, Brandt RMP, Melief CJM. Strict peptide length is not required for the indultion of cytotoxic T lymphocyte-mediated antiviral protection by peptide vaccination. Eur J Immunol 23: 1189-1192.

7. Combination treatment with Interleukin-2 and chemotherapeutic agents

ALBERT VON ROHR[1] and NICK THATCHER

1. Introduction

Most malignant tumours are still incurable in advanced stages. Surgery and radiotherapy certainly have an established role, but systemic treatment, usually chemotherapy, is considered standard treatment for disseminated malignancies. The activity of cytotoxic drugs is often unsatisfactory, and additional therapeutic options are clearly needed. Immunotherapy has emerged as a fourth modality for the treatment of certain malignant tumours [1] since recombinant materials became available for clinical use. Interleukin-2 (IL-2) is a cytokine which, when used as a single agent, showed activity against a range of tumours in both preclinical and clinical studies. More recently, IL-2 has been combined with chemotherapeutic drugs, and the number of studies investigating this approach is rapidly increasing. This review will summarise the clinical studies on IL-2 based chemoimmunotherapy published so far, but some general aspects concerning the combined use of IL-2 and chemotherapy will be considered first.

2. Combination of IL-2 and chemotherapeutic agents: general aspects

An additive or synergistic therapeutic effect between IL-2 (with or without additional LAK cells) and chemotherapeutic agents has been demonstrated in animal studies [2–10]. Moreover, IL-2 and cytotoxic drugs generally have different toxicity profiles, their antitumour effects are mediated by different mechanisms, and cultured or fresh multidrug-resistant human cancer cells usually maintain their susceptibility to IL-2 induced anti-tumour effectors [11–16]. These observations provide the rationale for the combined use of IL-2 and chemotherapeutic agents in the treatment of human malignancies. This approach does, however, require careful consideration of drug dosage,

[1] A. von Rohr is supported by the European Society for Medical Oncology (ESMO)

J. Wagstaff (ed.), The Role of Interleukin-2 in the Treatment of Cancer Patients, 95-121

scheduling, and sequence of administration in order to exploit possible additive or synergistic effects and to avoid undesirable interactions.

2.1. Mechanisms of action and interaction

The antitumour activity of IL-2 is assumed to be mainly mediated by immune effector cells, such as NK cells, LAK cells, cytolytic T lymphocytes and monocytes [17, 18]. The cytotoxicity of these effector cells can be induced, augmented, or maintained in vivo by treatment with IL-2 or ex vivo by incubation in IL-2. Treatment with ex vivo generated and adoptively transferred effectors (adoptive immunotherapy) requires the additional administration of systemic IL-2 to maintain their antitumour efficacy. In addition, IL-2 might induce humoral cytotoxicity by stimulating the production of tumour necrosis factor and other cytokines in certain cell populations. Moreover, it has been suggested that IL-2 has direct effects on tumour cells resulting in an increased susceptibility to cytotoxic agents [19], and IL-2 may even alter the vascular permeability in tumour tissues leading to an increased drug delivery and thus potentiate the effects of chemotherapy [20]. The clinical significance of the latter mechanisms is, however, uncertain. Furthermore, the pharmakokinetics of chemotherapeutic drugs may be altered after IL-2 treatment, but only few data on such drug interactions are available [21].

In contrast, the cytotoxicity of chemotherapeutic drugs is due to a direct tumour cell killing. Their effects on tumour cells may also include an alteration of cell membrane antigens or structure resulting in an increased susceptibility to immune lysis [22–24]. It has also been suggested that some forms of chemotherapy are able to arrest tumour cells in the G_0 or G_1 phase of the cell cycle when the cells are more susceptible to immune lysis [25]. In addition, most chemotherapeutic agents are capable of acting as immunomodulators. The majority of these drugs have immunosuppressive activity [26–28]; some can lead to immunosuppression as well as immunoaugmentation, depending on the dose (and schedule) used, and others have well established immunoaugmentative properties irrespective of the dose used. Chemotherapeutic agents may therefore be integrated into IL-2 based immunotherapy either for their cytotoxic potential, for their immunoaugmentative capacity, or for both.

2.2. Chemotherapeutic agents for cytoreduction

Chemotherapy with conventional doses and schedules of single cytotoxic drugs or multidrug regimens, aimed at reducing the tumour burden, may be combined with IL-2 based immunotherapy in order to exploit the efficacy of two different treatment modalities. In most studies using this approch, chemo- and immunotherapy have been administered sequentially rather than concomitantly. Tribute should be paid to the fact that prior immunosuppression may result in a temporary inability to generate cytolytic T lymphocytes; it may therefore be expedient to allow recovery from any agent with immunosuppressive effects before the immune system is stimulated with IL-2. In contrast to T lymphocytes, LAK cells do not, however, require a fully competent or intact immune system to mediate anti-tumour effects in vivo [29].

2.3. Chemotherapeutic agents for immunoaugmentation

Chemotherapeutic drugs can enhance a variety of immune functions by different mechanisms [30]. In some agents, several mechanisms may be involved at the same time. Modulating effects on the IL-2 dependent cell-mediated cytotoxicity are of special interest here, and they are briefly summarised for some cytotoxic agents frequently used in combination with IL-2.

An enhancing effect of low dose **cyclophosphamide** (CTX) on cell-mediated immunity has been demonstrated in many animal and human studies. The current hypothesis is that low dose CTX selectively inhibits the suppressor T cell function [31–33]. IL-2 is known to stimulate all subsets of T cells rather than simply the T helper and T cytolytic cells that one might want to be activated preferentially. Therefore low doses of CTX (50–350 mg/m^2) were given in human studies before IL-2 in an attempt to decrease T suppressor cell activity and to permit the proliferation and maturation of other subclasses of T cells, unimpeded by suppressor influences. In addition, CTX is capable of modulating nonspecific cell-mediated cytotoxicity. Serial measurements during treatment with low dose IL-2 in cancer patients, who had previously received a single CTX dose, showed that the maximum values for both NK and LAK activity were significantly greater in patients treated with low dose CTX (300 mg/m^2) than in patients treated with higher CTX doses (600 or 1200 mg/m^2) and in control patients [34]. It is evident from animal studies that the timing of IL-2 and CTX administration is crucial since maximum therapeutic efficacy was demonstrated only when IL-2 was given within 1 to 4 days after CTX [35]. Administration of LAK cells in addition to combined IL-2 and CTX did not result in a therapeutic benefit [6, 36].

Animal studies show that **doxorubicin** (DOX) augments the therapeutic effects of IL-2 [19, 37] and acts synergistically with IL-2 and LAK cells in adoptive immunotherapy [38]. DOX seems to improve the migration of LAK cells to tumour sites [5] and to enhance the cytolytic activity of T lymphocytes towards allogeneic and syngeneic tumour cells [39, 40]. Moreover, it has been suggested that DOX induces IL-2 release itself [41]. Animal and human studies demonstrated that neither the cytotoxicity of immune effector cells nor their generation is significantly inhibited by DOX [5, 42–45].

In vitro studies showed that **cisplatin** (DDP) in therapeutic doses is capable of stimulating killer monocytes for an enhancement of their cytotoxicity, with this effect not being due to inactivation of suppressor cells [46]. In animal studies, enhanced cytolytic activity of macrophages [47] and the release of interleukin-1 from peritoneal macrophages [48] have been observed after DDP administration. Consistent enhancement of these immune functions seems to occur in settings where DDP dosing is equivalent to therapeutic levels. In addition, DDP therapy is capable of augmenting endogenous NK cytotoxicity [49]. In vitro, DDP inhibits the generation of LAK effectors at high concentrations and causes an unresponsiveness to IL-2 which recovers spontaneously within 24 to 48 hours or after high doses of IL-2. In vivo, however, these inhibitory effects were not observed, most likely because the plasma concentrations were lower than that effective in the in vitro experiments, and subsequent LAK cell generation was not impaired [50, 51].

Exposure to **dacarbazine** (DTIC) can result in a significant induction of tumour cell immunogenicity. After DTIC treatment, murine lymphomas were found to be highly immunogenic and were rejected by immunocompetent animals [52–54]. Antigenic alterations, possibly due to DTIC-induced somatic mutations, have been suggested as the underlying mechanism of this phenomenon [55]. In vitro, these DTIC-treated cells were actually less susceptible to NK lysis; however, tumour rejection is likely to result from in vivo development of cytolytic T lymphocytes [56]. NK activity is not suppressed by DTIC in mice [43, 44]. In a human study it has recently been demonstrated that patients pretreated with standard doses of DTIC were still able to generate significant NK and LAK activities during subsequent IL-2 therapy [51].

2.4. Dosage and administration of IL-2

Some important points on IL-2 dosage and administration must be remembered before studies using this agent are compared. A wide range of IL-2 dosages and schedules, with or without additional LAK cells, has been clinically investigated in combination with chemotherapeutic agents. Consideration must be given to the fact that recombinant IL-2 is produced by several manufacturers, each product having its own specific activity. The IL-2 preparations most commonly used are those of the Cetus corporation and of Hoffmann-La Roche. In this review, all IL-2 doses are expressed as international units (IU). For comparison purposes, 1 Cetus unit equals 6 IU or 2.3 Roche units, and 1 Roche unit equals 2.6 IU.

The schedule of IL-2 administration is another point requiring attention. The maximally tolerated dose is considerably greater when IL-2 is given as bolus infusions than when given continuously [57]. For equivalent total doses, continuous IL-2 infusions result in greater biological effects as compared to bolus infusions ('bolus infusion' meaning a maximum administration time of 30 minutes) [58]. Accordingly, it has been demonstrated in many clinical studies that lower absolute IL-2 doses are sufficient for the induction of quantitatively similar biological effects when the drug is given continuously than when given as bolus infusions.

The multisystem toxicity profile of IL-2 is well defined. For a given IL-2 dosage and schedule of administration, the toxicity is largely predictable and may in fact be used for the definition of IL-2 dose levels. The following gradation has been employed in this review:

- **High dose IL-2** refers to a dose range ($\geq 50 \times 10^6$ IU/m²/d given as bolus infusion, or $\geq 15 \times 10^6$ IU/m²/d as continuous infusion for several consecutive days) which is likely to cause toxicities requiring intensive care support in a significant proportion of treated patients. IL-2 should not be given in this dose level unless regular access to intensive care facilities is available.
- **Moderate dose IL-2** indicates a dose range which does usually not cause such severe side effects, although the treatment normally requires hospitalisation on a regular oncology ward.
- **Low dose IL-2** indicates a dose range ($\leq 24 \times 10^6$ IU/m²/d given as bolus infusion, or $\leq 7 \times 10^6$ IU/m²/d as continuous infusion for several consecutive days) which can usually be given on an outpatient basis. Life-threatening side-effects are unlikely to occur; however, constitutional symptoms are common and dose-limiting for ambulatory patients.

3. Therapeutic studies

3.1. Malignant melanoma

Clinical trials demonstrated that low, albeit reproducible, response rates to various types of immunotherapy including IL-2 (with or without LAK cells) can be achieved in malignant melanoma (MM). Treatment with combined IL-2 and chemotherapeutic agents is best investigated in this tumour. Published therapeutic studies are summarised in Tables 1a and 1b.

3.1.1. Studies using IL-2 and chemotherapeutic agents without additional cytokines

Three studies have investigated IL-2 preceded by a single low dose of CTX for immunomodulation in patients with MM. In the study reported by Mitchell [59, 60], treatment consisted of CTX 350 mg/m² given as a bolus infusion, followed after 3 days by IL-2 in a dose of 21.6×10^6 IU/m² daily for 5 days on 2 successive weeks. At least 3 cycles of this treatment were given, separated by a rest period of 1 week, on an outpatient basis. In some patients, the IL-2 dose was increased up to 43.2×10^6 IU/m²/d during the second and third cycle. Nine responders, including 2 complete remissions, were observed in 38 patients (RR 24%). Sites of response included visceral metastases (both complete responders had liver involvement). The median duration of response was 9 months. Toxicity was well manageable, with 2 patients requiring an overnight hospitalisation.

A German multicentre trial, reported by Lindemann [61], employed the same design and schedule as in Mitchell's study. CTX was given at the same dose, and the IL-2 starting dose was 18×10^6 IU/m²/d bolus i.v. with escalation up to 36×10^6 IU/m²/d in subsequent cycles. The usual dose-dependent IL-2 toxicity was seen, but no patient, even when treated at the

Table 1a. Overview of clinical trials using combined IL-2 (± LAK cells) and chemotherapeutic agents in malignant melanoma

Author [Reference]	Study design	Evaluable patients	Number of patients with CR	Number of patients with PR	RR
Mitchell [60]	CTX i.v. d1 IL-2 low dose bolus i.v. d3–7/10–14 (dose escalation in some patients)	38	2	7	24%
Lindemann [61]	CTX i.v. d1 IL-2 low dose bolus i.v. d3–7/10–14 (dose escalation in some patients)	18	0	2	11%
Croghan [62]	CTX i.v. d1 IL-2 low dose bolus i.v. d4–8/11–15 (dose escalation)	25	0	0	0%
Rosenberg [63]	CTX i.v. d1 IL-2 high dose bolus i.v. d2–5 (or d2–7)	13	0	2	15%
Shiloni [64]	DTIC i.v. d1 IL-2 high dose cont. i.v. d4–9	18	2	2	22%
Dummer [65]	DTIC i.v. d1–5 IL-2 high dose cont. i.v. d21–24/28–31	14	0	5	36%
Dorreen [66]	DTIC i.v. d1–5 IL-2 high dose cont. i.v. d16–20/23–27	4 (study ongoing)	0	2	50%
Flaherty [69]	DTIC i.v. d1 IL-2 low dose bolus i.v. d15–19/22–26	32	1	6	22%
Papadopoulos [71]	DTIC i.v. d1–5 IL-2 low dose bolus i.v. d1–5/8–12	30	4	6	33%
Stoter [75]	IL-2 high dose cont. i.v. d1–5/12–17 DTIC i.v. d26 followed after 2 cycles by maintenance: alternating IL-2 × 5d/DTIC q21d	25	2	4	24%
Dillman [77]	IL-2 high dose cont. i.v. d1–5/11–15 LAK cells d10–13 DTIC i.v. d28(–30)	27	2	5	26%
Blair [78]	DDP and DTIC i.v. d1 IL-2 low dose bolus i.v. d12–16/19–23	28	5	7	43%
Demchak [80]	IL-2 high dose bolus i.v. d1–5/15–19 DDP (and WR-2721) i.v. d32 + 53	27	3	7	37%
Thatcher [84]	FAA i.v. d1 + 3 + 5 + 7 IL-2 intrasplenically d2 and i.v. (1-hr-infusions) d2 + 4 + 6 + 8	34	1	4	15%
Total		333	22	59	24%

Table 1b. Overview of clinical trials using combined IL-2 (± LAK cells), α-interferon, and chemotherapeutic agents in malignant melanoma

Author [Reference]	Study design	Evaluable patients	Number of patients with CR	Number of patients with PR	RR
Sznol [85, 86]	IL-2 moderate dose or high dose cont. i.v. d1–5/11–15 LAK cells (starting on d11) CTX i.v. d9 DOX i.v. d9 α-IFN s.c., starting on d21, 3 times weekly for 3 weeks (plus aspirin)	45	0	8	18%
Hamblin [87, 88]	DTIC i.v. d1 DDP i.v. d1 IL-2 high dose cont. i.v. d12–17/20–25 α-IFN s.c. d12–24 on alternate days	12	3	7	83%
Kirchner [89]	CBDCA i.v. d1 + 22 DTIC i.v. d1 + 22 IL-2 low dose s.c., starting on d36, 3 times weekly for 6 weeks α-IFN s.c., starting on d36, 3 times weekly for 6 weeks	22	1	7	36%
Richards [90]	BCNU i.v. d1 DTIC i.v. d1–3/22–24 DDP i.v. d1–3/22–24 IL-2 (dose?) bolus i.v. d4–8/17–21 α-IFN s.c. d4–8/17–21 Tamoxifen 2 × 10 mg/d p.o. for 6 weeks	25	6	9	60%
Total		104	10	31	39%

higher IL-2 dose levels, required admission to the intensive care unit (ICU). Two out of 18 evaluable MM patients, most of whom had received previous radio- or chemotherapy, achieved a partial remission (RR 11%). No complete remissions were, however, seen.

In a phase I/II study reported by Croghan [62], an IL-2 bolus dose of 21×10^6 IU/m²/d was chosen as the maximally tolerated dose, with fatigue, decreased performance status, weight gain, hypotension, and altered mental function being dose-limiting side effects. IL-2 was given daily for 5 days on 2 successive weeks, starting 4 days after a single dose of CTX (350 mg/m² i.v.), and cycles were repeated after 3 weeks. Neither complete nor partial remissions were seen in 25 melanoma patients, the best result being a mixed response in a patient with subcutaneous nodules. The authors compared this study to their previous experience with equivalent doses and administration of IL-2 alone and concluded that pretreatment with low dose CTX increased the toxicity without therapeutic benefit.

The Surgery Branch of the United States National Cancer Institute (NCI) probably has the most extensive experience worldwide in the use of high dose

IL-2, and its effectiveness in combination with escalating doses of CTX was investigated by one protocol. A recent update by Rosenberg [63] included 13 melanoma patients. Treatment consisted of a single intravenous CTX dose ranging from 10 to 50 mg/kg, followed after 24 to 36 hours by IL-2 given as bolus infusions in a dose of 600,000 IU/kg every 8 hours for 4 to 6 days. Only 2 partial remissions were achieved (RR 15%), and although the number of patients treated was small, it was concluded that an advantage of this regimen was unlikey as compared to IL-2 alone. Severe toxicities included weight gain of more than 10% (in 37% of all courses administered), hypotension requiring pressors (40%), thrombocytopenia $< 20{,}000/mm^3$ (20%), disorientation or coma (20%), mucositis requiring liquid diet (7%), and central line sepsis (13%).

In several other trials, IL-2 has been combined with dacarbazine (DTIC) which is generally considered the most active single chemotherapeutic agent in metastatic MM. Shiloni [64] reported on an ongoing international multicentre study in which DTIC 850 mg/m^2 i.v. was given on day 1, followed 3 days later by high dose IL-2 as a continuous infusion (18×10^6 $IU/m^2/d$) for 5 consecutive days. Thirty patients with progressing melanoma but reasonably good performance status were given up to 6 treatment cycles, the first two at 13-day intervals and further cycles at 20-day intervals. Four out of 18 evaluable patients responded (RR 22%), including 2 complete remissions. Sites of response included lung, spleen, skin, and lymph nodes. Nine patients received 3 or more cycles. Twenty five percent of the patients experienced severe weight gain (> 10%), and 15% required ICU admission.

Dummer [65] reported on a trial in which DTIC was given in a dose of 250 $mg/m^2/d$ as bolus infusions from day 1 to 5, alternating with 18×10^6 $IU/m^2/d$ of IL-2 administered as continuous infusions from day 21 to 24 and day 28 to 31. A new course was started on day 42. The usual side effects were seen, but weight gain was only mild due to a continuous furosemide infusion. A 36% remission rate was achieved in 14 previously untreated patients, but no complete responses were seen. An ongoing study with similar design was reported by Dorreen [66] in which melanoma patients are treated with DTIC 250 $mg/m^2/d$ from day 1 to 5 and IL-2 in a dose of 18×10^6 $IU/m^2/d$. IL-2 was administered as two 5-day continuous infusions from day 16 to 20 and day 23 to 27. Patients received at least 1 further course after a rest period of 1 week. Two out of 4 patients, who have completed the treatment so far, achieved a partial remission.

Other trials investigated DTIC with sequential low dose IL-2. In a phase I/II study reported by Flaherty [67–69], DTIC 1000 mg/m^2 was given as a 24-hour-infusion on day 1, followed after 2 weeks by bolus IL-2 in either of 3 dose levels (12, 18, or 24×10^6 $IU/m^2/d$). In addition, intrapatient dose escalations by 6×10^6 IU/m^2 were allowed in subsequent cycles unless grade III or IV toxicity occurred. IL-2 was given on an outpatient basis, and cycles were repeated after 28 days. Three cycles were given before responses were evaluated. A response rate of 22% was achieved, including 1 complete remission of a lung metastasis and 6 partial remissions in patients with lymph node, liver and lung disease. The median duration of response was 4.7 months. This regimen was generally well tolerated, with grade IV toxicity being restricted to granulocytopenia and thrombocytopenia. During the 127 treatment courses, 27 dose adjustments for IL-2 were necessary. Only 2 of 32 patients required hospitalisation as a result of treatment toxicity (1 patient required an overnight admission for hypotension and i.v. fluids but was able to continue daily treatment; 1 patient with upper gastrointestinal bleeding from a gastric ulcer with grade IV thrombocytopenia after DTIC).

In a phase I/II study performed at the M.D. Anderson Center [70, 71], treatment consisted of DTIC as a continuous infusion from day 1 to 5 (200 $mg/m^2/d$) and concomitant bolus IL-2 from day 1 to 5 and day 8 to 12 in one of 3 dose levels (12, 18, or 24 $\times$ 10^6 $IU/m^2/d$) with cycles being repeated after 4 weeks. The 30 study patients of fairly young age (median 45 years) and good performance status were treated on an outpatient basis. Three patients required temporary hospitalisation to continue treatment. The remission rate was 33% (4 CR, 6 PR) with responding sides including lung, pleura, liver, bone, spleen, lymph nodes, skin, and subcutaneous tissue.

In 2 trials, high dose IL-2 has been administered before DTIC. The multicentre study reported by Stoter [72–75] included 25 evaluable patients who were given 18 $\times$ 10^6 $IU/m^2/d$ of IL-2 as a continuous infusion from day 1 to 5 and day 12 to 17, followed by DTIC 850 mg/m^2 on day 26. This induction cycle was repeated once after 5 weeks. Maintenance therapy was scheduled 3 weeks after the completion of of the induction treatment and consisted of IL-2 given as continuous infusion in the same dose but for 5 days only, alternating with DTIC 850 mg/m^2 every three weeks, for a total of 18 weeks. Toxicity included constitutional symptoms in most patients, and 2 patients had a weight gain of more than 10%. Eight patients required admission to the ICU due to myocardial injury, ventricular tachycardia, sepsis, or hypotension and oliguria. In 3 patients, the study treatment was discontinued because of toxicity (myocardial injury, ventricular tachycardia, septic shock). The response rate was 24%. Two complete responders had lymph node metastases as the only site of disease, but partial remissions were seen in visceral sites as well. All responses occurred during the 2 induction cycles. None of the patients with more than 2 metastatic organ sites responded.

The study performed by the NBSG [76, 77] investigated high dose IL-2 in conjunction with LAK cells and sequential DTIC. Treatment consisted of an IL-2 priming cycle (18 $\times$ 10^6 $IU/m^2/d$ as continuous infusion) from day 1 to 5, followed by 4 days of leukapheresis for in vitro LAK cell generation, and then again continuous IL-2 for another 108 hours accompanied by reinfusion of the LAK cells during the first 3 days. DTIC treatment started on day 28 with a total of 1200 mg/m^2 being given as an intravenous infusion over 30 minutes to 4 hours either as a single dose or split over 2 or 3 days. There was no additive toxicity except for thrombocytopenia which delayed treatment in 2 out of 27 evaluable patients. One patient had myocardial ischaemia. Four patients required vasopressors for hypotension, and 5 patients required intermittent oxygen for dyspnoea. Severe side effects attributed to DTIC included granulocytopenia, diarrhoea, nausea, vomiting and anorexia requiring parenteral nutritional support. Two patients achieved a CR and 5 patients achieved a PR, for an overall remission rate of 26%, with a further three patients having mixed responses. The partial responses were brief, ranging from 1 to 6 months, whereas the complete responses have been sustained for 13+ and 24+ months.

Two therapeutic studies in which IL-2 has been combined with cisplatin (DDP) are of particular interest. Blair [78] reported a regimen consisting of DDP 100 mg/m^2 and additional DTIC 750 mg/m^2, both given on day 1. Low dose bolus IL-2 (24 $\times$ 10^6 IU/m^2/d) was administered on an outpatient basis from day 12 to 16 and day 19 to 23. This treatment was repeated after 4 weeks. The response rate of 43% (5 CR and 7 PR in 28 patients) was greater than in a group of patients with similar characteristics treated with high dose IL-2 ($\pm$ LAK cells) in a concurrent non-randomised trial (10% remission rate). Toxicity was less severe and median survival was better in the chemotherapy/IL-2 group than in the high dose IL-2 group (10.0+ months versus 5.5 months).

In the second study [79, 80], 27 evaluable patients were treated with bolus IL-2 at a dose of 600,000 IU/kg intravenously every 8 hours from day 1 to 5 and day 15 to 19, followed by high dose DDP in either of 2 regimens. The first 20 patients received 135 to 150 mg/m^2 together with 910 mg/m^2 of the chemoprotectant WR-2721 on days 32 and 53. Because of a considerable incidence (40%) of grade IV nephrotoxicity, predominantly in patients with liver metastases, this schedule was modified, and 7 subsequent patients received DDP 50 mg/m^2/d (without WR-2721) from day 32 to 34 and day 53 to 55. No significant nephrotoxicity was observed with this split administration. Severe IL-2 toxicities included myocarditis or subendocardial myocardial infarction (1 patient), weight gain of more than 10% (10 patients), hypotension requiring pressors (18 patients) and a persistent symmetric polyarthritis (2 patients). Transient elevation of creatinine occurred in 4 patients but never caused a delay in the administration of DDP. The overall response rate was 37%, and 3 complete remissions lasting 9, 16, and 30+ months were observed. Partial and complete responses were seen only in patients responding to IL-2. Tumour regressions (including minor responses) were noted after IL-2 treatment in 7 patients and after DDP administration in 14 patients, suggesting a noncrossresistance between the treatment components.

Flavone acetic acid (FAA) is a synthetic flavonoid known to have activity against a spectrum of murine solid tumours, to augment NK cytotoxicity, to induce interferon α/β, and to act synergistically with IL-2 in the treatment of murine renal cancer [81–83]. FAA is best considered a biological response modifier but may have some antiproliferative or cytotoxic activity as well [82]. In a study performed in our own institution [84], IL-2 has been employed in combination with FAA. Five doses of IL-2 were given, the first dose intrasplenically on day 1, a second dose 4 hours later intravenously, and further 3 doses intravenously on alternate days. IL-2 was administered over 1 hour at single doses of 66 $\times$ 10^6 IU/m^2. The day before each IL-2 treatment, patients received FAA at a dose of 4,800 mg/m² as a 6-hour-infusion. A new cycle was started on day 22, and a maximum of 3 courses were given to 34 patients. One complete and 4 partial remissions were observed (RR 15%). Responses occurred in pulmonary and hepatic metastases, but mainly in non-visceral sites, and response durations ranged from 3+ to 14 months. Toxicity was generally mild or moderate and always transient with no patient requiring intensive care facilities. Severe side effects included transient ventricular tachycardia (in a patient who was later shown to have myocardial metastases), grade IV leuco- and thrombocytopenia (in patients with bone marrow metastases), hypotension requiring fluid therapy, dyspnoea at rest, and central and peripheral neurotoxicity.

3.1.2. Studies using IL-2 and chemotherapeutic agents with additional α-interferon

Treatment of metastatic MM with α-interferon (α-IFN) is well documented, and reproducible remission rates of approximately 15% are achieved with this cytokine given as a single agent. Moreover, α-IFN shows synergism with IL-2 in preclinical models. As yet, α-IFN is the only additional cytokine which has been integrated into combinations of IL-2 and chemotherapeutic agents.

A trial reported by Sznol [85, 86] used IL-2 in conjunction with LAK cells and immunomodulatory doses of CTX and DOX. In a pilot evaluation, IL-2 was given as a moderate dose continuous infusion (7.8×10^6 IU/m²/d) from day 1 to 5 and day 11 to 15, and LAK cells on days 11, 12 and 14. The IL-2 dosage was increased to 15.6×10^6 IU/m²/d and the duration of LAK cell infusions reduced to 2 days for the phase II part of the study. Single doses of both CTX (300 mg/m²) and DOX (25 mg/m²) were given after leukapheresis on day 9. Treatment was then continued on day 21 with α-IFN (12×10^6 U/m² s.c. three times weekly) and aspirin (4×600 mg daily p.o.) for 3 weeks. Toxicity was moderate before and most severe after the IL-2 dose was increased. A response rate of 18%, with no complete remissions, was observed, with remissions in skin, lymph nodes, and lung but no other visceral sites. Remission durations were rather short, ranging from 3 to 10+ months (median <6 months).

Results from initial trials using platinum-containing regimens are more promising. Hamblin [87, 88] reported a regimen consisting of DDP 100 mg/m² and DTIC 750 mg/m² on day 1, followed after 12 days by concurrent high dose continuous infusion IL-2 (18×10^6 IU/m²/d) and subcutaneous α-IFN (3×10^6 U on alternate days) for 2 weeks. Courses were repeated after 28 days off treatment. Haematological toxicity was predominant. Ten remissions (3 CR, 7 PR) were seen in 12 patients (RR 83%). Two patients in complete remission had an early CNS relapse, but the third complete responder remains disease-free after 14 months. This study illustrates that the problem of CNS prophylaxis could become important with regimens yielding a high peripheral remission rate.

Kirchner reported on a study in which two doses of carboplatin (CBDCA; 400 mg/m²) and DTIC (750 mg/m²) were given on days 1 and 22, followed by a 6 week period of combination immunotherapy with low dose IL-2 and standard dose α-IFN, both given subcutaneously 3 times a week [89]. One complete and 7 partial remission were observed in 22 patients (RR 36%), and these responses were fairly durable (CR: 12+ months, PR: median 9+ months). The complete remission was seen in a patient with lung metastases, and partial responses were seen in lung, liver, spleen, soft tissue, skin, and lymph node secondaries. Thrombocytopenia after the chemotherapy was the predominant toxicity, but the long term immunotherapy was associated with significant cumulative constitutional symptoms. Response rate and remission duration was better in this study than in a previous trial with IL-2 and α-IFN alone conducted by the same institution.

Preliminary results of a study reported by Richards [90] show a 60% response rate (6 CR, 9 PR) for a regimen consisting of BCNU 150 mg/m^2 on day 1, DTIC 220 mg/m^2/d and DDP 25 mg/m^2/d from day 1 to 3 and day 22 to 24 each. This chemotherapy was accompanied by immunotherapy with bolus infusion IL-2 and subcutaneous α-IFN, both given from day 4 to 8 and day 17 to 21, and by hormone therapy with tamoxifen 20 mg daily p.o. for 6 weeks. Unfortunately, the IL-2 dose remains unclear as the product used is not specified, and no details on the toxicity of this treatment are reported. Median response duration has not been reached after 5 months.

3.2. Renal cell cancer

Renal cell cancer (RCC) has attracted some enthusiasm for investigating IL-2 in combination with chemotherapy (see Table 2) as this tumour, like MM, is responsive to IL-2 based immunotherapy.

Several studies used IL-2 in combination with variable doses of CTX. Three trials which have been outlined in section 3.1.1. also contained patients with RCC, but none of 30 patients showed a response [61–63]. In a phase I study performed at the Memorial Sloan-Kettering Cancer Center in New York [91, 92], CTX at low doses (50 or 350 mg/m^2) was given intravenously on day 1, followed by 6×10^6 IU/m^2/d of IL-2 as an intravenous 6-hour-infusion from day 5 to 9 and day 12 to 16. Thereafter, IL-2 treatment was continued by subcutaneous administration 5 times a week with weekly 33% dose increments. Three out of 7 patients with RCC achieved a response; no details are given for response parameters such as sites and durations. The authors state that rebound lymphocytosis, cytotoxicity against NK-sensitive target cells, and antitumour efficacy of this regimen were enhanced as compared to one of their previous trials employing intermittent IL-2 alone.

The study by Sznol using IL-2 in conjunction with LAK cells, low dose CTX, and DOX, followed by α-IFN and aspirin (described in section 3.1.2.), reported a 23% response rate (partial remissions only) in 35 evaluable patients with RCC [85, 86]. Tumour regressions were predominantly seen in lung metastases, but also in lymph node and bone secondaries. The RCC patients had more durable remissions, ranging from 4+ to 13+ months, than the

Table 2. Overview of clinical trials using combined IL-2 and chemotherapeutic agents in renal cell carcinoma

Author [Reference]	Study design	Evaluable patients	Number of patients with		RR
			CR	PR	
Lindemann [61]	CTX i.v. d1 IL-2 low dose bolus i.v. d3–7/10–14 (dose escalation in some patients)	14	0	0	0%
Croghan [62]	CTX i.v. d1 IL-2 low dose bolus i.v. d4–8/11–15 (dose escalation)	13	0	0	0%
Rosenberg [63]	CTX i.v. d1 IL-2 high dose bolus i.v. d2–5 (or d2–7)	3	0	0	0%
Kolitz [91]	CTX i.v. d1 IL-2 i.v. (6-hr-infusion) d5–9/12–16; subsequently s.c. 5 times/week with weekly 33% dose increments	7	Responses in 3 patients		43%
Sznol [85, 86]	IL-2 moderate dose or high dose cont. i.v. d1–5/11–15 LAK cells (starting on d11) CTX i.v. d9 DOX i.v. d9 α-IFN s.c., starting on d21, 3 times weekly for 3 weeks (plus aspirin)	35	0	8	23%
Pinto [93]	IL-2 low dose bolus i.v. d1–4/8–11 VBL i.v. d5 + 12	10	0	0	0%
Bar [94]	IL-2 high dose cont. i.v. d1–5/12–16 VBL i.v. d24 + 26	12	1	3	33%
Total		94	15		16%

melanoma patients treated in the same study.

In two studies, IL-2 has been combined with vinblastine (VBL) which is one of the most active chemotherapeutic drugs in RCC. In the study reported by Pinto [93] bolus IL-2 (24×10^6 IU/m²/d) was given from day 1 to 4 and day 8 to 11, and VBL (5 mg/m²) on days 5 and 12. Treatment was repeated every 21 days. The best results were 3 minor responses, but no partial or complete remissions were seen in 10 patients who completed a minimum of 3 courses. The most frequent significant toxicities were fatigue, hypotension, nausea/vomiting and bone marrow suppression. Five of 43 cycles were administered with delay. One patient only required an IL-2 dose reduction, and 79% of the VBL dose intended in the protocol could be given.

In the study reported by Bar [94], IL-2 was given as a high dose continuous infusion (18×10^6 IU/m²/d) from day 1 to 5 and day 12 to 16, followed by VBL 4 mg/m² on days 24 and 26. Treatment was repeated after 35 days, and patients were evaluated after 2 cycles. Responding patients continued therapy for up to 6 cycles. In 12 evaluable patients who had fairly good prognostic factors (performance status 0 or 1, no systemic pretreatment), a response rate of 33% was seen including 1 CR (5+ months) and 3 PR (9+, 10+, and 11+ months). Two patients with PR are free of disease after resection of persistent renal primary lesions. Sites of response were renal primary, renal bed, lymph nodes, lung, liver, and bone lesions. Toxicity was substantial; therapy was aborted in 3 patients because of grade IV toxicity, and another 4 patients required an IL-2 dose reduction.

3.3. Colorectal cancer

Studies in patients with colorectal cancer are summarised in Table 3. One trial already mentioned in section 3.1.1. [62] investigated low dose bolus IL-2 following a single low dose of CTX but yielded no objective responses in 8 evaluable patients. Treatment regimens in other trials were based upon IL-2 and 5-fluorouracil (5-FU), the latter being the agent considered standard chemotherapy in advanced colorectal cancer.

Table 3. Overview of clinical trials using combined IL-2 and chemotherapeutic agents in colorectal cancer

Author [Reference]	Study design	Evaluable patients	Number of patients with		RR
			CR	PR	
Croghan [62]	CTX i.v. d1 IL-2 low dose bolus i.v. d4–8/11–15 (dose escalation)	8	0	0	0%
Hiddemann [95]	IL-2 high dose cont. i.v. d1–5 5-FU (plus leucovorin) cont. i.v. d8–10	22	0	3	14%
Hamblin [96]	IL-2 high dose cont. i.v. d1–5 5-FU bolus i.v. d7 + 14 + 21	7	0	2	29%

Hiddemann [95] reported on a phase II study in patients with progressive metastatic colorectal cancer who had failed previous chemotherapy with 5-FU and leucovorin. Treatment consisted of a 5-day high dose continuous IL-2 infusion (18×10^6 IU/m²/d), followed after a rest period of 2 days by 5-FU 600 mg/m²/d with leucovorin 300 mg/m²/d, both given continuously for another 3 days. After a minimum of 2 courses, a partial remission was achieved by 3 of 22 evaluable patients (RR 14%), and a minor response or a stable disease was seen in another 5 patients. This study indicates that tumours refractory to 5-FU/leucovorin may still be responsive to the combination of these agents with IL-2. Toxicity was substantial with a complete discontinuation of treatment being required in 4 patients, and IL-2 doses having to be reduced in 24% of the treatment courses administered.

In the phase II study reported by Hamblin [96], 7 previously untreated patients with good performance status (KP ≥80) and progressive metastatic or unresectable colorectal cancer (Dukes stage C or D) were treated with high dose continuous IL-2 (18×10^6 IU/m²/d) from day 1 to 5, followed by 5-FU 600 mg/m² by intravenous bolus infusions on days 7, 14, and 21. Treatment was repeated on day 28, and efficacy was assessed after 2 courses. A maximum of 6 cycles was administered. Two partial remissions and 3 stable diseases were noted in 7 patients. Toxicity was substantial with all patients having hypotension and oliguria. Disorientation and severe weight gain (> 10%) were seen in 2 patients. One patient died from perforation of the bowel at the site of the carcinoma, and a second patient suffered from pulmonary embolism during the IL-2 infusion.

3.4. Breast cancer

Two studies are published and summarised in Table 4. Three heavily pretreated patients with breast cancer were included in the NCI trial investigating CTX followed by high dose bolus IL-2 (study outlined in section 3.1.1.). None of them achieved a remission [63]. Another trial has been reported by Paciucci [45]. Four patients with particularly adverse prognostic characteristics (inflammatory breast cancer refractory to radiotherapy and to DOX containing regimens, bulky tumours) were treated with high dose continuous IL-2 (20.4×10^6 IU/m²/d) for 6 days; DOX 30 mg/m² was given 24 hours after discontinuation of IL-2, and IL-2 infusions were resumed 24 hours after chemotherapy. The intended total treatment time was 28 days, with 4 DOX doses. However, no patient received the fourth dose because of toxicity, mainly neutropenia and thrombocytopenia. Three out of the 4 patients exhibited tumour regressions of more than 50%, but regrowth was observed within 1 week after interrupting treatment, and these responses therefore do not qualify for true partial remissions. The fourth patients had a minor response.

Table 4. Overview of clinical trials using combined IL-2 and chemotherapeutic agents in breast cancer

Author [Reference]	Study design	Evaluable patients	Number of patients with		RR
			CR	PR	
Rosenberg [63]	CTX i.v. d1 IL-2 high dose bolus i.v. d2–5 (or d2–7)	3	0	0	0%
Paciucci [45]	IL-2 high dose cont. i.v. d1–6/8–13/15–20/22–27 DOX i.v. d7 + 14 + 21 + 28	4	0	0	0%

3.5. Head and neck cancer

Two phase I/II studies are published (see Table 5) and both of them used DDP and 5-FU with sequential IL-2. The study reported by Valone [97] included 5 patients (no details on pretreatment, histology and localisation of tumours are given in this preliminary report). Treatment consisted of high dose DDP 100 mg/m² on days 1 and 8, 5-FU 1000 mg/m²/d as a continuous infusion from day 1 to 3, and bolus low dose IL-2 daily from day 15 to 19, with cycles being repeated after 28 days. The IL-2 dose was escalated, but the maximum tolerated dose (MTD) was found to be in the low dose range (12×10^6 IU/m²/d), with hypotension, fluid overload, leukopenia, thrombocytopenia, renal toxicity, ototoxicity, anorexia and weight loss being dose-limiting. Ninety four percent of the DDP dose intensity intended in the protocol, and 73% of the IL-2 dose intensity, could actually be delivered. Responses were noted in 3 patients.

Table 5. Overview of clinical trials using combined IL-2 and chemotherapeutic agents in head and neck cancer

Author [Reference]	Study design	Evaluable patients	Number of patients with		RR
			CR	PR	
Valone [97]	DDP i.v. d1 + 8 5-FU cont. i.v. d1–3 IL-2 low dose bolus i.v. d15–19	5	Responses in 3 patients		60%
Dimery [98]	DDP i.v. d1 5-FU cont. i.v. d1–4 IL-2 low/moderate dose (dose escalation) bolus i.v. d3–6/9–13	20	1	6	35%

In the second trial, reported by Dimery from the M.D. Anderson Cancer Center [98], DDP 100 mg/m² was given on day 1 and 5-FU 1000 mg/m²/d as a continuous infusion from day 1 to 4. IL-2 was given as bolus infusions from day 3 to 6 and day 9 to 13 of each 28-day cycle, with doses being escalated from 3 to 36×10^6 IU/m²/d. In this study, the MTD for IL-2 was 24×10^6 IU/m²/d with hypotension and cardiotoxicity (arrhythmias, ischemia) being dose-limiting. A maximum of 6 cycles (median 3) was given to 25 patients. One complete (8+ months) and 6 partial remissions were observed in 20 evaluable patients (RR 35%).

3.6. Gastric cancer

The studies in gastric cancer are summarised in Table 6. Merrouche published a phase II trial comprising patients with metastatic or unresectable gastric cancer most of whom had prior chemotherapy or radiotherapy [99]. Treatment consisted of high dose BCNU (800 mg/m²) followed by autologous bone marrow transplantation and, starting 24 hours after the graft, a continuous infusion of IL-2 at 18 × 10^6 IU/m^2/d for at least 6 days. No patient had IL-2 for longer than 8 days as toxicity was prohibitive. In 14 patients evaluable for response, 1 complete (21 months) and 2 partial remissions were achieved (RR 21%). Sites of response were unresectable primary, liver and lymph node metastases.

Table 6. Overview of clinical trials using combined IL-2 and chemotherapeutic agents in gastric cancer

Author [Reference]	Study design	Evaluable patients	Number of patients with		RR
			CR	PR	
Merrouche [99]	BCNU high dose i.v. with ABMT IL-2 high dose cont. i.v. × 6–8 days	14	1	2	21%
Akiyoshi [100]	MMC or DOX i.v. d1 IL-2 (dose?) bolus i.v. d4–8	10	0	6	60%

Akiyoshi reported on a trial which, amongst others, included 10 patients with advanced gastric cancer for whom standard therapy had failed [100]. Treatment comprised a single dose of mitomycin C (MMC; 12 mg/m^2) or DOX (25 mg/m^2) on day 1 followed by IL-2 as bolus infusions every 12 hours from day 4 to 8 (unfortunately the source of IL-2 used is not specified, and therefore the dose level remains unclear). Severe toxicity was not encountered. Six partial remissions and 5 minor responses were seen in 21 evaluable study patients, and all PR occurred in patients with gastric cancer, amounting to a RR of 60% in this tumour.

3.7. Lung cancer

So far only a limited number of patients with both non-small cell lung cancer (NSCLC) and small cell lung cancer (SCLC) has been included in studies using IL-2 in combination with chemotherapy (see Table 7). The study reported by Paciucci [45] which has already been described in section 3.4. (weekly DOX and high dose continuous IL-2) included 8 patients with NSCLC resistant to previous chemotherapy and radiotherapy. As mentioned, this regimen proved to be unfeasible because of toxicity. No patient was able to tolerate this treatment for 4 weeks as intended in the protocol. Notwithstanding, partial remissions were seen in 2 patients and minor responses in another 2 patients. The study reported by Valone [97] which has been mentioned in section 3.5. also included 20 patients with NSCLC. This treatment with high dose DDP on days 1 and 8, continuous infusion 5-FU from day 1 to 3, and bolus low dose IL-2 from day 15 to 19 yielded a RR of 35% in NSCLC.

Preliminary results of an ongoing CALGB study in SCLC have been reported by Clamon [101]. So far, 67 patients with previously untreated

Table 7. Overview of clinical trials using combined IL-2 and chemotherapeutic agents in lung cancer

Author [Reference]	Tumour	Study design	Evaluable patients	Number of patients with		RR
				CR	PR	
Paciucci [45]	NSCLC	IL-2 high dose cont. i.v. d1–6/8–13/15–20/22–27 DOX i.v. d7 + 14 + 21 + 28	8	0	2	25%
Valone [97]	NSCLC	DDP i.v. d1 + 8 5-FU cont. i.v. d1–3 IL-2 low dose bolus i.v. d15–19	20	Responses in 7 patients		35%
Clamon [101]	SCLC	DDP/DOX/CTX/VP-16 × 4 cycles followed in pts. with PR/NC/PD by IL-2 moderate dose cont. i.v. d1–4 weekly	10 (study ongoing)	2*	1*	30%*

* Responses to IL-2 only

extensive SCLC have been accrued into this phase II study, and they were treated with 4 cycles of the conventional PACE chemotherapy regimen containing DDP, DOX, CTX, and VP-16. In patients with partial remission, stable or progressive disease, treatment was then continued after a rest period of 4 weeks with moderate dose IL-2 (11.7×10^6 IU/m^2/d) given as a continuous infusion for 96 hours. This IL-2 therapy was repeated weekly for a total of 4 courses prior to reevaluation. Finally, patients with a complete remission to IL-2 received 2 additional courses, and those with a partial remission received 4 additional IL-2 courses. Ten patients who have completed the IL-2 treatment are evaluable so far, and objective responses to IL-2 were observed in 3 out of these 10 patients (2 complete remissions, 1 regression of evaluable disease). Dose-limiting toxicities required discontinuation of IL-2 treatment in 7 patients, and IL-2 was stopped in 2 additional patients because they developed brain metastases (one of these patients had a regression of chest and liver lesions). During the PACE chemotherapy, 3 patients developed congestive heart failure preventing IL-2 treatment. These data suggest that IL-2 has activity in SCLC and can induce further tumour regression after combination chemotherapy with PACE. The results for the many patients still under therapy are awaited with interest.

3.8. *Other trials*

A few trials in other tumour types remain to be mentioned, as well as studies including patients with a variety of different tumours in which treatment results are not specified for each tumour type. These studies are summarised in Table 8.

Table 8. Other trials using combined IL-2 and chemotherapeutic agents

Author [Reference]	Tumour	Study design	Evaluable patients	Number of patients with		RR
				CR	PR	
Favrot [102]	Neuro-blastoma	High dose chemoradiotherapy with ABMT IL-2 high dose cont. i.v. d1–5/12–16 × 2 cycles, followed by maintenance	4	1*	1*	50%*
Kawata [104]	Hepato-cellular carcinoma	Randomisation after surgery: • DOX i.a. d8 post op. plus IL-2 low dose for 3 weeks (start 10 days post op.) plus spleen-derived LAK cells • DOX i.a. d8 post op.	12 12	Adjuvant setting (see text)		
Dave [105]	Colorectal and breast cancer	CTX single dose p.o.; followed after 10 days by IL-2 low dose cont. i.v. d1–4 weekly for 4 weeks, and α-IFN i.m. 3 × weekly for 4 weeks; followed by 5-FU (plus leucovorin) bolus i.v. d1–5 q21d × 4	18	1	3	22%
Dave [105]	Melanoma, renal cell cancer, sarcomas and other solid tumours	CTX single dose p.o.; followed after 10 days by IL-2 low dose cont. i.v. d1–4 weekly for 4 weeks (on alternate weeks thereafter), and α-IFN i.m. 3 × weekly for 4 weeks (on alternate weeks thereafter)	20	0	2	10%
Akiyoshi [100]	Various solid tumours other than gastric cancer	MMC or DOX i.v. d1 IL-2 (dose?) bolus i.v. d4–8	11	0	0	0%
Kolitz [91]	Various tumours other than RCC	CTX i.v. d1 IL-2 i.v. (6-hr-infusion) d5–9/12–16; subsequently s.c. 5 times/week with weekly 33% dose increments	17	Responses in 3 patients		18%
Oldham [106]	Various solid tumours	CTX i.v. d1 IL-2 × 5d (no details available)	39	0	2	5%

* Responses to IL-2 only

A trial reported by Favrot indicates that chemoresistant **neuroblastoma** is potentially sensitive to immunotherapy with IL-2 [102]. The study included 4 children, aged between 5 and 7 years, who were in partial remission after induction therapy (including surgery) when they received 2 cycles, 3 months apart, of myeloablative chemoradiotherapy with BCNU/VM-26/carboplatin, and vincristine/melphalan/total body irradiation, respectively. Each cycle was followed by an autologous bone marrow transplantation. The patients had persistent active disease, but a normal brain CT scan, 75 to 120 days after the second autograft when IL-2 treatment was started. High dose IL-2 was given in a dosage of 18×10^6 IU/m²/d as a continuous infusion for 120 hours, and after a rest period of 6 days the treatment was resumed and given for another 108 hours in the same dosage. This induction course was repeated once after a 3-week interval. Finally, after a rest of 4 weeks, one IL-2 maintenance course was given at the same dose, but for 120 hours only. Responders to IL-2 treatment included 1 patient with a complete remission of bone metastases and local abdominal tumour lasting for 9 months before the disease relapsed at the site of the primary abdominal lesion. A second patient had a partial remission of bone marrow metastases (with normalisation of urinary catecholamine metabolites) lasting for 6+ months. Stable and progressive disease was seen in 1 patient each. These patients were carefully monitored and given prophylactic antibiotics. IL-2 toxicity was transient and not life-threatening despite the heavy pretreatment. Although 3 of the 4 patients had abnormal haematological parameters, especially a low platelet count, before initiation of the IL-2 treatment, the haematological toxicity was moderate. Red cell transfusions were required by 3 patients but platelet transfusions by 1 patient only. In a separate report [103], the authors present another neuroblastoma patient who received the same treatment except for an allogeneic non T cell-depleted (instead of an autologous) bone marrow transplantation. In this patient, the reversible reactivation of an acute graft-versus-host disease was seen during the IL-2 infusion.

Preliminary results of an interesting study were reported by Kawata [104]. Patients, after radical surgery for **hepatocellular carcinoma**, were randomised to receive an adjuvant treatment with either DOX, IL-2, and spleen-derived LAK cells (group A), or DOX alone (group B). Eight days after surgery, a single dose of 20 mg DOX was given to all patients as an arterial infusion. Patients in group B were followed without any further therapy until recurrence, whereas additional immunotherapy was given to patients in group A. Starting on day 10 after surgery, 3 infusions of spleen-derived LAK cells were administered in conjunction with IL-2 in a very low dose of 3.5×10^5 IU/d for 3 weeks. Unfortunately, no details on the administration of IL-2 and LAK cells are given in this preliminary report. Twelve patients are evaluable in each of the 2 treatment groups. After 1 year, the respective disease free rate was 85% for group A and 68% for group B, and the respective survival rate was 100% for group A and 89% for group B. No severe toxicity was encountered.

Dave reported on a continuing study [105] in which 28 patients with

colorectal or breast cancer were treated with a single low dose of CTX (350 mg/m² p.o.), followed 10 days later by low dose IL-2 given as a continuous infusion for 4 days weekly, with concomitant α-IFN 9 × 10^6 U/m² i.m. 3 times weekly, both for 4 weeks. This immunotherapy was then followed by a chemotherapy consisting of 5-FU 375 mg/m²/d and leucovorin 500 mg/m²/d, both agents given as bolus infusions for 5 consecutive days and repeated after 3 weeks for a total of 4 cycles. One complete, 3 partial, and 1 minor response were seen in 18 evaluable patients, but these responses were not specified for tumour types. The same report [105] also included 30 patients with **MM, RCC, sarcomas, and other solid tumours**. This population received the same initial treatment as mentioned above, however, instead of 5-FU/leucovorin, the immunotherapy with IL-2 and α-IFN was continued on alternate weeks. Two out of 20 evaluable patients achieved a partial remission, and 1 patient had a minor response (again not specified for tumour types). In both patient groups, the treatment was given on an outpatient basis but no details concerning patient characteristics and response quality are available.

The study reported by Akiyoshi [100] mentioned in section 3.6. also included 11 evaluable patients with various (unspecified) advanced **solid tumours other than gastric cancer** for which standard therapy had failed. Treatment consisted of bolus IL-2 (dosage unclear) for 5 days preceded by a single low dose of MMC or DOX. In contrast to patients with gastric cancer, no objective remissions were seen in other tumour types, the best result being a minor response.

The Memorial Sloan-Kettering phase I study of low dose CTX followed by escalating doses of IL-2 has already been summarised in section 3.2. [91]. Besides the RCC patients mentioned, 17 patients with various advanced **solid tumours other than RCC** were also treated, and three achieved an objective remission (RR 18%). Responses are not specified by tumour type, and no details were given for response qualities.

Preliminary results of an ongoing phase II trial conducted by the National Biotherapy Study Group in patients with **various advanced solid tumours** have been reported by Oldham [106]. Treatment consisted of 2 cycles with CTX 1000 mg/m² followed by IL-2 for 5 days (no details on the administration schedule of IL-2 are given). Stable and responding patients then received another 4 cycles with IL-2 alone. In 39 evaluable patients, most of them having received systemic pretreatment, 2 partial remissions were seen in patients with prostate cancer and breast cancer, and 2 out of 8 patients with MM had minor responses.

4. Conclusions and perspectives

The clinical studies conducted so far have demonstrated that arguably better therapeutic results are seen in certain tumours with the combination of IL-2 and chemotherapeutic agents than with either component used alone. Particularly encouraging results have been reported in MM. Interesting activities have also been seen in gastric cancer, head and neck cancer, and neuroblastoma, whereas the results in RCC are rather disappointing. In malignancies other than MM, however, larger patient numbers will have to be treated and randomised studies are required to assess the significance of IL-2 based chemoimmunotherapy.

In patients with MM, it has been shown that durable remissions in non-visceral as well as visceral metastatic sites can be induced. DDP and analogues proved to be the most promising chemotherapeutic agents in combination with IL-2, and the therapeutic efficacy seems to be even better by using additional α-IFN. These data suggest that the integration of additional cytokines into IL-2 based chemoimmunotherapy could be a promising approach. The respective contribution of single agents will, however, only be elucidated by appropriate trials.

IL-2 treatment with high doses show no clear advantage over lower doses. Therefore, an important task seems to be the development of chemoimmunotherapy regimens suitable for an outpatient setting, with IL-2 being given by infusion pumps or by subcutaneous self-administration.

So far, most therapeutic studies have been undertaken in patients with bulky disease. There is, however, some preclinical evidence that immunotherapy may be most effective in situations with low tumour burden [107, 108]. Initial debulking chemotherapy with induction of a maximal tumour response, followed by IL-2 based treatment, may be an approach well worth investigating, particularly under the aspect that several clinical trials confirmed the preclinical finding that multidrug-resistant tumour cells generally remain susceptible to the cytolytic activity of IL-2 dependent immune effector cells. Indeed several studies are in progress or have been reported in a preliminary fashion in which IL-2 treatment is given to patients with minimal residual disease or in an adjuvant setting [101, 104, 109]. The long term results of these trials are awaited with interest.

References

1. Oldham R. Biotherapy: The fourth modality of cancer treatment. J Cell Physiol 1986; 4(Suppl): 91–9.
2. Papa MZ, Yang JC, Vetto JT, et al. Combined effects of chemotherapy and interleukin 2 in the therapy of mice with advanced pulmonary tumors. Cancer Res 1988; 48: 122–9.
3. LoRusso PM, Aukerman SL, Polin L, et al. Antitumor efficacy of interleukin-2 alone and in combination with adriamycin and dacarbazine in murine solid tumor systems. Cancer Res 1990; 50: 5876–82.
4. Silagi S, Schaefer AE. Successful immunotherapy of mouse melanoma and sarcoma with recombinant interleukin-2 and cyclophosphamide. J Biol Response Mod 1986; 5: 411–22.
5. Wiltrout RH, Salup RR. Adoptive immunotherapy in combination with chemotherapy for cancer treatment. Prog Exp Tumor Res 1988; 32: 128–53.
6. Kedar E, Ben-Aziz R, Shiloni E. Therapy of advanced solid tumors in mice using chemotherapy in combination with interleukin-2 with and without lymphokine-activated killer cells. Isr J Med Sci 1988; 24: 494–504.
7. Hosokawa M, Yabiku T, Ikeda J, et al. Effects of a combination of cyclophosphamide and human recombinant interleukin 2 on pulmonary metastasis after the surgical removal of a 3-

methylcholanthrene-induced primary tumor in autochthonous mice. Jpn J Cancer Res(Gann)1988; 79: 1147–54.
8. Hosokawa M, Sawamura Y, Morikage T, et al. Improved therapeutic effects of interleukin 2 after the accumulation of lymphokine-activated killer cells in tumor tissue of mice previously treated with cyclophosphamide. Cancer Immunol Immunother 1988; 26: 250–6.
9. Eggermont AMM, Sugarbaker PH. Efficacy of chemoimmunotherapy with cyclophosphamide, interleukin-2 and lymphokine activated killer cells in an intraperitoneal murine tumour model. Br J Cancer 1988; 58: 410–4.
10. Eggermont AMM, Sugarbaker PH. Augmentation of antitumor effects of intraperitoneal (ip) interleukin-2 (IL-2) by monoclonal antibodies (MoAbs) and cyclophosphamide (CY). Proc AACR 1989; 30: 376 (# 1493).
11. Gambacorti-Passerini C, Radrizzani M, Erba E, et al. Lysis by activated lymphocytes of melanoma and small cell lung cancer cells surviving in vitro treatment with mafosfamide. Cancer Res 1987; 47: 2547–52.
12. Gambacorti-Passerini C, Rivoltini L, Supino R, et al. Susceptibility of chemoresistant murine and human tumor cells to lysis by interleukin 2-activated lymphocytes. Cancer Res 1988; 48: 2372–6.
13. Allavena P, Grandi M, D'Incalci M, et al. Human tumor cell lines with pleiotropic drug resistance are efficiently killed by interleukin-2 activated killer cells and by activated monocytes. Int J Cancer 1987; 40: 104–7.
14. Allavena P, Damia G, Colombo T, et al. Lymphokine-activated killer (LAK) and monocyte-mediated cytotoxicity on tumor cell lines resistant to antitumor agents. Cell Immunol 1989; 120: 250–8.
15. Schroit AJ, Fidler IJ. The use of activated macrophages for the destruction of heterogeneous metastasis. In: Horn KV, Powers WE, Sloane BF, editors. Mechanisms of cancer metastasis: Potential therapeutic implications. Boston: M. Nijhoff, 1986: 207–26.
16. Harker WG, Tom C, McGregor JR, et al. Human tumor cell line resistance to chemotherapeutic agents does not predict resistance to natural killer or lymphokine-activated killer cell-mediated cytolysis. Cancer Res 1990; 50: 5931–6.
17. Mulé JJ, Yang JC, Lafreniere R, et al. Identification of cellular mechanisms operational in vivo during the regression of established pulmonary metastases by the systemic administration of high-dose recombinant interleukin 2. J Immunol 1987; 139: 285–94.
18. Mertelsmann R, Welte K. Restorative immunotherapy with interleukin-2. In: Reif AE, Mitchell MS, editors. Immunity to cancer. Orlando: Academic Press, 1985: 485–97.
19. Ades EW, McKemie CR III, Wright S, et al. Chemotherapy subsequent to recombinant interleukin-2 immunotherapy: Protocol for enhanced tumoricidal activity. Nat Immun Cell Growth Regul 1987; 6: 260–8.
20. Mitchell MS. Biomodulation: A classification and overview. In: Reif AE, Mitchell MS, editors. Immunity to cancer. Orlando: Academic Press, 1985: 401–11.
21. Chabot GG, Flaherty LE, Valdivieso M, Baker LH. Alteration of dacarbazine pharmakokinetics after interleukin-2 administration in melanoma patients. Cancer Chemother Pharmacol 1990; 27: 157–60.
22. Schlager SI. Relationship between cell mediated and humoral immune attack on tumour cells. I. Drug and hormonal effects on susceptibility to killing and macromolecular synthesis. Cell Immunol 1981; 58: 398–414.
23. Schlager SI. Relationship between cell mediated and humoral immune attack on tumour cells. II. The role of cellular lipid metabolism and cell surface charge in the outcome of immune attack. Cell Immunol 1982; 66: 300–16.
24. Borsos T. Induction of tumour immunity by intratumoral chemotherapy. Ann N Y Acad Sci 1976; 276: 565–80.
25. Mathé G. Effectiveness of murine leukemia chemotherapy according to the immune status. Cancer Immunol Immunother 1977; 2: 139–41.
26. Braun DP, Harris JE. Modulation of the immune response by chemotherapy. Pharmacol Ther

1981; 14: 89–122.
27. Kempf RA, Mitchell MS. Effects of chemotherapeutic agents on the immune response. I. Cancer Invest 1984; 2: 459–66.
28. Kempf RA, Mitchell MS. Effects of chemotherapeutic agents on the immune response. II. Cancer Invest 1985; 3: 23–33.
29. Mulé JJ, Shu S, Rosenberg SA. The anti-tumor efficacy of lymphokine-activated killer cells and recombinant interleukin 2 in vivo. J Immunol 1985; 135: 646–52.
30. Mastrangelo MJ, Berd D, Maguire H Jr. The immunoaugmenting effects of cancer chemotherapeutic agents. Semin Oncol 1986; 13: 186–94.
31. Berd D, Mastrangelo MJ. Effect of low dose cyclophosphamide on the immune system of cancer patients: Reduction of T-suppressor function without depletion of the CD8+ subset. Cancer Res 1987; 47: 3317–21.
32. Berd D, Maguire HC Jr, Mastrangelo MJ. Impairment of concanavalin A-inducible suppressor activity following administration of cyclophosphamide to patients with advanced cancer. Cancer Res 1984; 44: 1275–80.
33. Glaser M. Augmentation of specific immune response against a syngeneic SV40-induced sarcoma in mice depleted of suppressor T cells with cyclophosphamide. Cell Immunol 1979; 48: 339–45.
34. Eiseman J, Melink T, Bell M, et al. Determination of an optimal immunomodulatory dose for cyclophosphamide in combination with interleukin-2. Proc AACR 1989; 30: 378 (# 1501).
35. Kedar E, Ben-Aziz R, Epstein E, Leshem B. Chemoimmunotherapy of murine tumors using interleukin-2 (IL-2) and cyclophosphamide. IL-2 can facilitate or inhibit tumor growth depending on the sequence of treatment and the tumor type. Cancer Immunol Immunother 1989; 29: 74–8.
36. Kedar E, Chriqui-Zeira E, Kyriazis AP. Immunotherapy of murine and human tumors in mice with lymphokines and interleukin-2 propagated lymphocytes. J Biol Response Mod 1984; 3: 517–26.
37. Yu PP, Paciucci PA, Holland JF. Activity of human recombinant interleukin-2 (rIL-2) and doxorubicin in tumour-bearing BL/6 mice. Proc AACR 1986; 27: 317 (# 1258).
38. Salup RR, Back TC, Wiltrout RH. Successful treatment of advanced murine renal cell cancer by bicompartemental adoptive chemoimmunotherapy. J Immunol 1987; 138: 641–7.
39. Ehrke MJ, Ryoyama K, Cohen SA. Cellular basis for adriamycin-induced augmentation of cell-mediated cytotoxicity in culture. Cancer Res 1984; 44: 2497–2504.
40. Ehrke MJ, Ryoyama K, Mihich E. Generation of cytotoxic lymphocytes in cultures of spleen cells from tumor bearing mice: Modification by adriamycin and cyclophosphamide treatment of the mice. Proc AACR 1981; 22: 273.
41. Ehrke MJ, Maccubbin D, Ryoyama K, et al. Correlation between adriamycin-induced augmentation of interleukin 2 production and of cell-mediated cytotoxicity in mice. Cancer Res 1986; 46: 54–60.
42. Kempf RA, Cebul RA, Mitchell MS. Antitumour effects of doxorubicin against a virally-induced rat osteosarcoma with minimal immunosuppression. J Immunopharmacol 1980; 2: 509–25.
43. Mantovani A, Luini W, Peri G, et al. Effect of chemotherapeutic agents on natural cell-mediated cytotoxicity in mice. J Natl Cancer Inst 1978; 61: 1255–61.
44. Spreafico F. Heterogeneity of the interaction of anticancer agents with the immune system and its possible relevance to chemoimmunotherapy. Oncology 1980; 37(Suppl 1): 9–18.
45. Paciucci PA, Holland JF, Ryder JS, et al. Immunotherapy with interleukin-2 by constant infusion with and without adoptive cell transfer and with weekly doxorubicin. Cancer Treat Rev 1989; 16(Suppl A): 67–81.
46. Kleinerman ES, Zwelling LA, Muchmore AV. Enhancement of naturally occurring human spontaneous monocyte-mediated cytotoxicity by cis-diamminedichloroplatinum(II). Cancer Res 1980; 40: 3099–3102.
47. Sodhi A, Bhatia P. In vitro activation of murine macrophages and their increased capacity to

lyse target cells after cisplatin treatment. Indian J Exp Biol 1986; 24: 565–72.
48. Gupta P, Sodhi A. Increased release of interleukin-1 from mouse peritoneal macrophages in vitro after cisplatin treatment. Int J Immunopharmacol 1987; 9: 385–8.
49. Lichtenstein AK, Pende D. Enhancement of natural killer cytotoxicity by cis-diamminedichloroplatinum (II) in vivo and in vitro. Cancer Res 1986; 46: 639–44.
50. Allavena P, Pirovano P, Bonazzi C, et al. In vitro and in vivo effects of cisplatin on the generation of lymphokine-activated killer cells. J Natl Cancer Inst 1990; 82: 139–42.
51. Redman BG, Flaherty L, Chou TH, et al. Sequential dacarbazine/cisplatin and interleukin-2 in metastatic melanoma: Immunological effects of therapy. J Immunother 1991; 10: 147–51.
52. Contessa AR, Bonmassar A, Giampietri A, et al. In vitro generation of a highly immunogenic subline of L1210 leukemia following exposure to 5-(3,3'-Dimethyl-1-triazeno)imidazole-4-carboxamide. Cancer Res 1981; 41: 2476–82.
53. Nicolin A, Bini A, Coronetti E, Goldin A. Cellular immune response to a drug-treated L5178Y lymphoma subline. Nature 1974; 251: 654–5.
54. Bonmassar E, Bonmassar A, Vadlamudi S, Goldin A. Immunological alteration of leukemic cells in vivo after treatment with an antitumor drug. Proc Natl Acad Sci USA 1970; 66: 1089–95.
55. Fioretti MC, Bianchi R, Romani L, Bonmassar E. Drug-induced immunogenic changes of murine leukemia cells: Dissociation of onset of resistance and emergence of novel immunogenicity. J Natl Cancer Inst 1983; 71: 1247–51.
56. Franco P, Veronese F, Levi F, et al. Antibody-dependent cellular cytotoxicity against drug-induced antigens in L5178Y mouse lymphoma. Br J Cancer 1982; 46: 173–9.
57. Kohler PC, Hank JA, Moore KH, et al. Phase I clinical trial of recombinant interleukin-2: A comparison of bolus and continuous intravenous infusion. Cancer Invest 1989; 7: 213–23.
58. Thompson JA, Lee DJ, Lindgren CG, et al. Influence of dose and duration of infusion of interleukin-2 on toxicity and immunomodulation. J Clin Oncol 1988; 6: 669–78.
59. Mitchell MS, Kempf RA, Harel W, et al. Effectiveness and tolerability of low-dose cyclophosphamide and low-dose intravenous interleukin-2 in disseminated melanoma. J Clin Oncol 1988; 6: 409–24.
60. Mitchell MS, Kempf RA, Harel W, et al. Low-dose cyclophosphamide and low-dose interleukin-2 for malignant melanoma. Bull N Y Acad Med 1989; 65: 128–44.
61. Lindemann A, Hoeffken K, Schmidt RE, et al. A multicenter trial of interleukin-2 and low-dose cyclophosphamide in highly chemotherapy-resistant malignancies. Cancer Treat Rev 1989; 16(Suppl A): 53–7.
62. Croghan M, Hersh EM, Taylor C, et al. Phase I–II study of low dose cytoxan and recombinant interleukin-2 (IL-2) for the treatment of disseminated carcinoma. Proc ASCO 1989; 8: 180 (# 699).
63. Rosenberg SA, Lotze MT, Yang JC, et al. Experience with the use of high-dose interleukin-2 in the treatment of 652 cancer patients. Ann Surg 1989; 210: 474–85.
64. Shiloni E, Pouillart P, Janssens J, et al. Sequential dacarbazine chemotherapy followed by recombinant interleukin-2 in metastatic melanoma. A pilot multicentre phase I–II study. Eur J Cancer Clin Oncol 1989; 25(Suppl 3): S45–S49.
65. Dummer R, Becker J, Schulz A, et al. DTIC and sequential IL-2 for metastatic malignant melanoma. Eur J Cancer 1991; 27(Suppl 2): S153 (# 919).
66. Dorreen MS, Sreenivasan T, Bruce L, et al. Biological responses in patients undergoing interleukin-2 therapy for metastatic melanoma and renal cell carcinoma. Proc ASCO 1990; 9: 192 (# 744).
67. Flaherty L, Redman B, Chabot G, et al. Combination of dacarbazine (DTIC) and interleukin-2 (IL-2) in metastatic malignant melanoma (MMM). Proc ASCO 1988; 7: 254 (# 983).
68. Flaherty L. The combination of recombinant interleukin-2 and dacarbazine (DTIC) in metastatic malignant melanoma. Cancer Treat Rev 1989; 16(Suppl A): 65–6.
69. Flaherty LE, Redman BG, Chabot GG, et al. A phase I–II study of dacarbazine in combination with outpatient interleukin-2 in metastatic malignant melanoma. Cancer 1990; 65: 2471–7.

70. Papadopoulos NEJ, Howard J, Murray JL, et al. Phase I-II DTIC and interleukin-2 (IL-2) trial for metastatic malignant melanoma. Proc ASCO 1989; 8: 290 (# 1130).
71. Papadopoulos NEJ, Howard JG, Murray JL, et al. Phase II DTIC and interleukin 2 (IL-2) trial for metastatic malignant melanoma. Proc ASCO 1990; 9: 277 (# 1072).
72. Stoter G, Shiloni E, Gundersen S, et al. Alternating recombinant human interleukin-2 (rIL-2) and dacarbazine (DTIC) in metastatic melanoma. Proc ASCO 1989; 8: 281 (# 1095).
73. Stoter G, Shiloni E, Gundersen S, et al. Alternating recombinant human interleukin-2 and dacarbazine in advanced melanoma. A multicentric phase II study. Cancer Treat Rev 1989; 16(Suppl A): 59–63.
74. Stoter G, Shiloni E, Aamdal S, et al. Sequential administration of recombinant human interleukin-2 and dacarbazine in metastatic melanoma. A multicentre phase II study. Eur J Cancer Clin Oncol 1989; 25(Suppl 3): S41–S43.
75. Stoter G, Aamdal S, Rodenhuis S, et al. Sequential administration of recombinant human interleukin-2 and dacarbazine in metastatic melanoma: A multicenter phase II study. J Clin Oncol 1991; 9: 1687–91.
76. West W, Tauer K, Barth N, et al. Adoptive immunotherapy and sequential DTIC chemotherapy in metastatic melanoma. Proc ASCO 1989; 8: 281 (# 1094).
77. Dillman RO, Oldham RK, Barth NM, et al. Recombinant interleukin-2 and adoptive immunotherapy alternated with dacarbazine therapy in malignant melanoma: A National Biotherapy Study Group trial. J Natl Cancer Inst 1990; 82: 1345–9.
78. Blair S, Flaherty L, Valdivieso M, Redman B. Comparison of high dose interleukin-2 (HD IL-2) with combined chemotherapy/low dose IL-2 (chemo/IL-2) in metastatic malignant melanoma. Proc ASCO 1991; 10: 294 (# 1031).
79. Atkins M, Demchak P, Mier J, et al. Phase II study of alternating interleukin-2 (IL-2) and cisplatin (cisDDP) with WR-2721 in metastatic melanoma. Proc ASCO 1989; 8: 287 (# 1119).
80. Demchak PA, Mier JW, Robert NJ, et al. Interleukin-2 and high-dose cisplatin in patients with metastatic melanoma: A pilot study. J Clin Oncol 1991; 9: 1821–30.
81. Wiltrout RH, Boyd MR, Back TC, et al. Flavone-8-acetic acid augments systemic natural killer cell activity and synergizes with IL-2 for treatment of murine renal cancer. J Immunol 1988; 140: 3261–5.
82. Hornung RL, Young HA, Urba WJ, Wiltrout RH. Immunomodulation of natural killer cell activity by flavone acetic acid: Occurrence via induction of interferon α / β. J Natl Cancer Inst 1988; 80: 1226–31.
83. Urba WJ, Longo DL, Lombardo FA, Weiss RB. Enhancement of natural killer activity in human peripheral blood by flavone acetic acid. J Natl Cancer Inst 1988; 80: 521–5.
84. Thatcher N, Dazzi H, Mellor M, et al. Recombinant interleukin-2 (rIL-2) with flavone acetic acid (FAA) in advanced malignant melanoma: A phase II study. Br J Cancer 1990; 61: 618–21.
85. Sznol M, Clark J, Smith J, et al. A pilot evaluation of interleukin-2 (IL-2) and lymphokine activated killer (LAK) cells in combination with chemotherapy and alpha-interferon. Proc ASCO 1989; 8: 191 (# 742).
86. Sznol M, Clark J, Smith J, et al. A phase II study of IL-2/LAK in combination with chemotherapy and interferon-alfa in patients with metastatic melanoma and renal cell carcinoma (RCC). Proc ASCO 1990; 9: 196 (# 759).
87. Hamblin TJ, Davies B, Sadullah S, et al. A phase II study of the treatment of metastatic malignant melanoma with a combination of dacarbazine, cis-platin, interleukin-2 (IL-2) and alfa-interferon (IFN). Proc ASCO 1991; 10: 294 (# 1029).
88. Hamblin TJ, Davies B, Sadullah S, et al. A phase II study of the treatment of metastatic malignant melanoma with a combination of dacarbazine, cis-platin, interleukin-2 (IL-2) and alfa-interferon (IFN). Eur J Cancer 1991; 27(Suppl 2): S157 (# 939).
89. Kirchner H, Poliwoda H, Atzpodien J. Recombinant interleukin-2 and interferon-α in combination with carboplatin and DTIC in progressive metastatic melanoma. Eur J Cancer 1991; 27(Suppl 2): S157 (# 942).
90. Richards JM, Priest E, Hamasaki V, et al. Sequential chemoimmunotherapy for metastatic

melanoma. Proc ASCO 1991; 10: 298 (# 1046).
91. Kolitz JE, Merluzzi VJ, Welte K, et al. A phase I trial of recombinant interleukin-2 (rIL-2) and cyclophosphamide (CPM) in advanced malignancy. Proc ASCO 1986; 5: 235 (# 921).
92. Kolitz JE, Wong GY, Welte K, et al. Phase I trial of recombinant interleukin-2 and cyclophosphamide: Augmentation of cellular immunity and T-cell mitogenic response with long-term administration of rIL-2. J Biol Response Mod 1988; 7: 457–72.
93. Pinto HA, Yahanda A, Reese J, et al. Chemoimmunotherapy with recombinant interleukin-2 (rIL-2) and vinblastine (VBL) in metastatic renal cell carcinoma. Proc ASCO 1991; 10: 179 (# 579).
94. Bar MH, Valone FH, Rayner AA, et al. A phase I–II trial of combined interleukin-2 and vinblastine for metastatic renal cell carcinoma. Proc ASCO 1990; 9: 146 (# 568).
95. Hiddemann W, Ruelfs C, Ottensmeier C, et al. Combination of interleukin 2 with 5-fluorouracil and folinic acid in refractory colorectal cancer. Eur J Cancer 1991; 27(Suppl 2): S93 (# 540).
96. Hamblin TJ, Inzani V, Sadullah S, et al. A phase-II trial of recombinant interleukin-2 and 5-FU chemotherapy in patients with metastatic colorectal carcinoma. Cancer Treat Rev 1989; 16(Suppl A): 163–7.
97. Valone FH, Gandara DR, Deisseroth A, et al. Interleukin-2 (IL-2) combined with high-dose cisplatin (HDCP)/5-fluorouracil (5-FU) in metastatic non-small cell lung (NSCLC) and head and neck cancer. Proc ASCO 1989; 8: 194 (# 755).
98. Dimery I, Martin T, Bradley E, et al. Phase I trial of interleukin-2 (rIL-2) plus cisplatin (CDDP) and 5-fluorouracil (5-FU) in recurrent or advanced squamous cell carcinoma of the head and neck. Proc ASCO 1989; 8: 170 (# 660).
99. Merrouche Y, Negrier S, Rebattu P, et al. A phase II study of interleukin 2 (IL2) following high dose BCNU and autologous bone marrow transplantation (ABMT) in the treatment of metastatic gastric cancer. Proc ASCO 1991; 10: 161 (# 510).
100. Akiyoshi T, Arinaga S, Karimine N, et al. Effect of recombinant interleukin 2 in combination with mitomycin C or adriamycin on advanced cancer. Proc AACR 1990; 31: 273 (# 1616).
101. Clamon G, Goutsou M, Perry MC, et al. Interleukin-2 (IL-2) in extensive small cell lung cancer: A preliminary suggestion of activity. Proc ASCO 1991; 10: 267 (# 925).
102. Favrot MC, Michon J, Floret D, et al. Interleukin 2 immunotherapy in children with neuroblastoma after high-dose chemotherapy and autologous bone marrow transplantation. Pediatr Hematol Oncol 1990; 7: 275–84.
103. Favrot MC, Floret D, Negrier S, et al. Systemic interleukin-2 therapy in children with progressive neuroblastoma after high dose chemotherapy and bone marrow transplantation. Bone Marrow Transplant 1989; 4: 499–503.
104. Kawata A, Uchino J, Une Y, et al. Early postoperative chemoimmunotherapy with adriamycin, rIL-2 and spleen-derived LAK for hepatocellular carcinoma patients. Proc AACR 1991; 32: 251 (# 1490).
105. Dave HPG, Goldberg SL, Conde M, et al. Outpatient low-dose interleukin-2 with or without 5-fluorouracil/leucovorin for solid tumors. Proc ASCO 1991; 10: 217 (# 729).
106. Oldham RK, Stark J, Barth N, et al. Treatment of advanced cancers with cytoxan (CTX) and interleukin-2 (rIL-2): a phase II study. Proc AACR 1990; 31: 268 (# 1587).
107. Eggermont AMM, Marquet RL, De Bruin RWF, Jeekel J. Effects of the interferon inducer ABPP on colon cancer in rats; importance of tumor load and tumor site. Cancer Immunol Immunother 1986; 22: 217–22.
108. Greenberg PD, Klarnet JP, Kern DE, Cheever MA. Therapy of disseminated tumors by adoptive transfer of specifically immune T cells. Prog Exp Tumor Res 1988; 32: 104–27.
109. Gottlieb DJ, Brenner MK, He H, et al. A phase I clinical trial of recombinant interleukin 2 following high dose chemo-radiotherapy for haematological malignancy: Applicability to the elimination of minimal residual disease. Br J Cancer 1989; 60: 610–5.

8. Interleukin-2, lymphocytes and monoclonal antibodies

REINDER L.H. BOLHUIS and GERRIT STOTER

1. Introduction

The search for tumour specific immune reactions was triggered by the formulation of the immune surveillance hypothesis as early as 1909 [1] and by its later updates [2]. The central idea of immune surveillance is that the immune system has the capacity, not only to distinguish 'self' from 'non-self', but also to distinguish cancer cells in the body from their normal counterparts. As a result the immune system may arrest or eliminate the cancer cells from the tumour bearing host. The fascination with this concept has initiated and stimulated cancer immunologists to classify tumours on the basis of their antigenic 'make-up' and their reaction to cytokines. To this end a wide range of animal species were immunised with (human) tumour cells to raise antisera for the serological dissection of cancer. With the advent of monoclonal antibodies (mAb) an even more precise knowledge was gained about carbohydrate epitopes on the glycoprotein, glycolipid and ganglioside antigen structure of tumour cells [3]. All these efforts have generated serological reagents, that are now widely applied in the laboratory and clinic, ranging from application in fundamental tumour cell biology to the use for immunodiagnosis in the laboratory and *in vivo* and for immunotherapy.

Until recently it was not possible to characterise T-cell defined tumour associated antigens (TAA). Immunotherapy itself has become a major focus in the field of tumour immunology aiming at the development of effective anti-cancer treatment.

In this chapter we will focus attention on the basic mechanisms of the cellular immune system with antigens and tumour cells in particular. The specific receptors involved in specific recognition and delivering of the first signal for activation of immune cells will be described. The importance of costimulatory molecules involved in delivering a second signal to the T cell necessary for immune cell proliferation and differentiation into effector cells will also be illustrated. Finally, we will address the role of cytokines, interleukin-2 (IL-2) in particular, and their pleiotropic role in the immune system, on the major lymphocyte populations that mediate anti-tumour responses, and on how use is

J. Wagstaff (ed.), The Role of Interleukin-2 in the Treatment of Cancer Patients, 123-140.

being made of this knowledge for the design of antitumour therapeutic strategies based on these immunologic mechanisms and principles.

2. T and B lymphocytes

2.1. Introduction

Together T and B lymphocytes are able to recognise and respond to any possible micro-organism or foreign molecule or antigen. Their broad response is based on the high specificity and diversity of the immune system. Because of this high specificity and its ability to discriminate between 'self' and 'non-self', the immune system rarely mounts attacks on the body's normal tissues. The recognition of antigens by the B and T lymphocytes is mediated by specific receptors expressed on their surface and these membrane T cell receptor (TCR) and B cell antibody (Ab) receptor are strikingly similar in structure. The T lymphocytes respond to antigen recognition and binding by the secretion of molecules: lymphokines. Lymphokines facilitate the communication with other lymphocytes and leucocytes, and maintain their own state of activation, activate other immune cell populations and promote their proliferation. Within the T cell compartment different lymphocyte subsets exist, such as the T-helper cells and cytotoxic T lymphocytes (CTL). T-helper cells primarily produce lymphokines such as IL-2 and express the CD4 molecule on their surface. CTL make direct, specific contact with infected or cancer cells, secrete toxic molecules to kill them and express the CD8 molecule on their surface. Such tumour-specific immune responses by T lymphocytes are restricted by the major histocompatibility complex (MHC), i.e. (tumour-)antigens are specifically presented to them by MHC-class molecules on the target cells.

Tumour cells can also be killed following Ab binding to the tumour cell. The Ab is produced by B cells which recognise antigen via their membrane bound immunoglobulin (Ig), in a MHC-unrestricted fashion. Following Ab binding to the target cell complement factors can bind to it, and this complement pathway becomes activated resulting in complement dependent cytolysis (CDC) of the tumour cell. Alternatively, the Ab bound to the tumour cell can be recognised by receptors on various immune cells by its Fc-part. These Fc-receptors are expressed on, e.g., Natural Killer (NK) lymphocytes, monocytes, granulocytes or macrophages. This mechanism of target cell lysis is called Antibody Dependent Cellular Cytotoxicity (ADCC).

Finally, tumour cells can also directly be killed by NK cells and IL-2 activated T lymphocytes but in a MHC-unrestricted fashion. The MHC-unrestricted cytolysis of tumour cells by these immune lymphocytes involves multiple lymphocyte surface receptors. The varying combinations of these receptors provide the MHC-unrestricted cytolytic activity with tumour cell selectivity [for review 4, 5]).

2.2. Antigen specific receptors on B lymphocytes: immunoglobulin or antibody

An important feature of the antigen-specific immune system is its memory capacity. Once it has encountered and responded to an antigen it will respond upon antigen rechallenge in a much faster and more vigorous way. In the case of B cells, the primary response results in the production of IgM Ab, followed by the production of IgG class Ab, whereas the memory response always involves the production of IgG class Ab. Upon antigen binding the B cells become activated and this results in clonal expansion and differentiation into plasma cells that secrete large amounts of Ab with a single specificity. IL-2 plays a keyrole in this process, because it promotes not only the proliferation and maintenance of the activated state of $CD4^+$ helper T cells involved in Ab production, but it also promotes the proliferation and the differentiation of the B cells. An Ab produced by the progenitors of a single stimulated B cell, which has differentiated in an Ab-secreting plasma cell, is called mAb. Köhler and Milstein [6] developed a technique to immortalise B cells by the somatic hybridisation of B cells to 'immortal' tumour B cells. The resulting hybrid plasma cell secreting Ab thus has inherited the unlimited growth capacity and Ab producing ability of their respective parent cells.

This hybridoma technology has revolutionised immunology research. For instance, it opened the way to the development of a mAb based diagnosis and immunotherapy of cancer. These mAb based immunotherapy protocols have so far been focused on using them upon conjugation to effector compounds, such as bacterial or plant toxins, radio-nucleotides or cytotoxic drugs. However, this approach encountered problems, e.g. less biologic activity of the Ab due to the chemical coupling procedures or non-specific interactions of the Fc-parts of the Ab with Fc-receptors on cells of the reticular endothelial system, leading to their sequestration. The result of these interactions was the unwanted homing of the conjugated Ab in organs, such as liver and spleen, or the rapid clearance from the body.

2.3. The antigen specific T cell receptors

The T lymphocyte structures capable of specific antigen recognition are the membrane expressed polymorphic TCR [7, 8]. The polymorphic TCR are noncovalently associated with the nonpolymorphic CD3 signal transducing complex. Similar to B cells, the interaction of the TCR with an antigen, following target cell binding, results in the delivery of an activation signal to the T cell. In the case of a CTL, this results in delivery of a lethal hit to the target cell due to the secretion of cytotoxic molecules by these CTL. Subsequently the effector-target cell conjugate dissociates, the target cell disintegrates, and the CTL is capable of another attack on a tumour cell, so called recycling. The vast majority of antigen-specific T lymphocytes expresses the TCR$\alpha\beta$ receptor and are either of the $CD4^+$ or $CD8^+$ phenotype, as described earlier. The CD4 on the T-helper lymphocytes interacts with MHC class II molecules on the target cell, whereas the $CD8^+$ on CTL interacts with MHC class I on the target cells (MHC-restriction) [for review 9] (Figure 1).

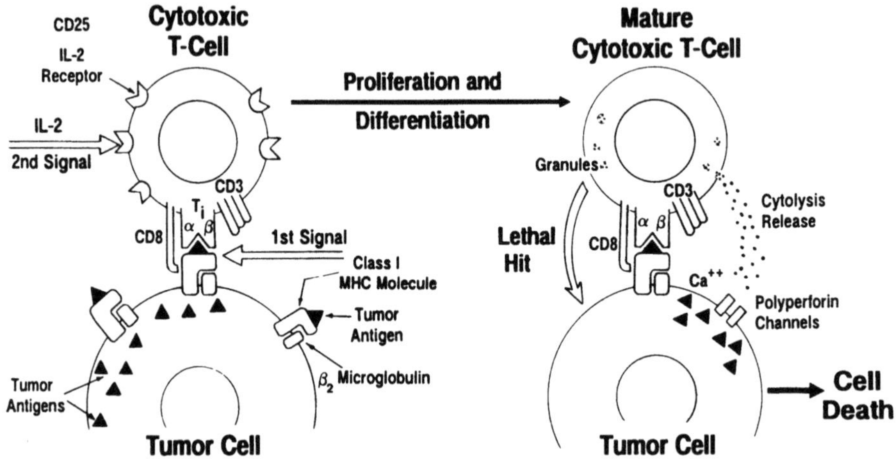

Figure 1. Recognition and killing by $CD8^+$ cytotoxic T cells.

A minor fraction of the TCR lymphocytes expresses the $\gamma\delta$ receptor and lacks the expression of the CD4 and CD8 antigens [10–15]. The gene organisation of the $TCR\gamma\delta$ is homologous to that of the $TCR\alpha\beta$. It has been suggested that $TCR\gamma\delta$ lymphocytes can also exert antigen-specific MHC-restricted antigen recognition [16–21], but recent evidence demonstrated that they are also capable of MHC-unrestricted 'superantigen' recognition [21, 22].

3. Lymphocyte populations exerting MHC-unrestricted cytolysis

3.1. Natural killer (NK) lymphocytes

Originally, MHC-unrestricted, 'spontaneous' cytolysis of tumour cells by lymphocytes was described as NK activity. This NK activity was exerted by lymphoid cells that have now been characterised as $TCR^-/CD3^-$ lymphocytes. As a consequence their lytic activity is, by definition, MHC-unrestricted and this feature reflects the critical difference to the antigen-specific, MHC-restricted $\alpha\beta/CD3^+$ T cell mediated cytolysis [9, 23, 24]. MHC-unrestricted cytolysis therefore represents an activity, not a cell population. MHC-unrestricted lysis has been termed earlier in the literature as 'nonspecific', 'anomalous', 'promiscuous', 'activated killer', 'natural killer-like', 'lymphokine activated killer' activity. It is directed against a wide variety of target cells including (autologous) tumour and virus infected cells [25–30; for review 4].

Another conclusion that can be drawn from the fact that NK lymphocytes lack the expression of the TCR$\alpha\beta$ or $\gamma\delta$ is that non-TCR structures must be involved in the MHC-unrestricted cytolytic process. However, 'classic' TCR$\alpha\beta$ lymphocytes as well as TCR$\gamma\delta$ lymphocytes are capable of exerting MHC-unrestricted lysis following appropriate activation with IL-2 [14, 21, 22]. This demonstrates that the precursor cells of lymphocytes with LAK activity are heterogeneous [4, 5], as has been already suggested by studies demonstrating that lymphocytes generated in mixed leucocyte culture were different from MHC-restricted CTL [25, 31–33]. An important notion is that the MHC-unrestricted lytic activity of lymphocytes shows no memory response.

What lymphocyte surface molecules are then involved in MHC-unrestricted lysis of tumour cells?

3.2. Lymphocyte membrane structures involved in MHC-unrestricted cytolysis

A key question is which lymphocyte surface molecules participate in the binding to and the subsequent MHC-unrestricted lysis of tumour target cells. Secondary to that question is whether the distinct lymphocyte subsets identified employ the same recognition and/or adhesion and signal-transducing molecules. We have already outlined in some detail that specific antigen recognition is mediated via the polymorphic receptors on B and T cells. It initiates a cascade of biochemical events that are essential to T cell activation [34]. Multiple lymphocyte surface molecules have meanwhile been identified which are capable of costimulation, resulting in the full activation of T and NK lymphocytes. The number of costimulatory molecules has already increased to more than twenty [for review 35]. In order to investigate T cell stimulation via the TCR and via costimulatory molecules, we made use of mAbs specific for CD3 or adhesion costimulatory structures on the lymphocytes. The assumption is that mAb mediated activation of T cells mimics the activity of the natural ligand for the lymphocyte cell surface molecules, i.e. TCR-antigen interactions. Three receptor ligand pathways have been characterised in detail:

- the CD2 Lymphocyte Function associated Antigen (LFA-3)
- LFA-1-InterCellular Adhesion Molecule (ICAM) and
- CD28-B7.

The adhesion molecules are the structures on lymphocytes which inform the cell that contact with a target cell has been made, either for the purpose of intercellular communication or target cell destruction. We know now that many of the adhesion molecules also mediate T and NK lymphocyte receptor costimulation and thus can be considered as messengers of information [14, 36–40, for review 41] (Figure 2). A further expansion of our understanding of receptor costimulation of lymphocytes involved the study of ligands which are extracellular matrix (ECM), on the T lymphocyte and which react with the opposing target cell. The receptors on the T lymphocytes mediating adhesion to the ECM are members of the Very Late Antigen (VLA or CD29) subfamily of integrins [for review 42]). The functional interplays between TCR and these distinct adhesion or activation sites make it clear that the response of T cells is very versatile: they allow the fine regulation of the immune response. The expression, function, and interplay of all these types of lymphocyte surface molecules is modulated by the action of lymphokines and vice versa. This implies that administration of even a single lymphokine such as IL-2 has multiple effects on lymphocyte activation, differentiation, traffic and homing. Moreover, these effects are not only influenced by what type of lymphokine is administered, but also by its dose level and the route of administration to the host.

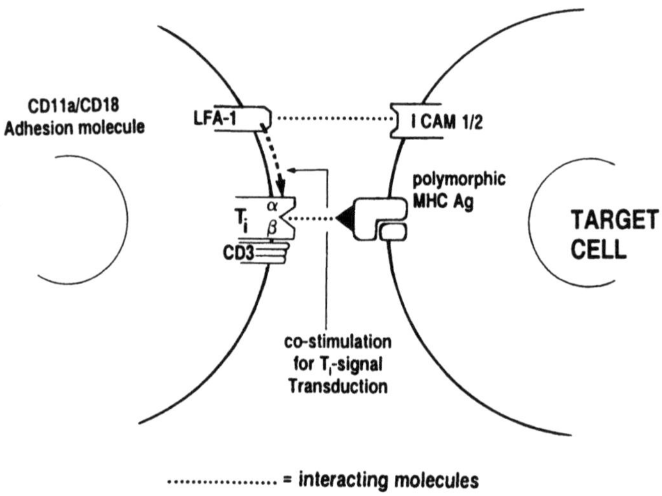

Figure 2. Adhesion molecules such as CD11a/CD18 (LFA-1) deliver costimulatory signals to the CD3-TCR complex following binding of their ICAM 1/2 counter structure.

4. Tumour specific antigens and tumour associated antigens (TAA)

For almost 50 years it has been known that chemically induced tumour cells express immunogenic antigens, as was demonstrated by tumour transplantation experiments [43]. The hallmark of the tumour rejection antigens of inbred mice is their individual distinctiveness. That means that a chemically induced tumour of a particular histologic type will not crossreact with another tumour, even when induced by the same chemical (carcinogen) and in the same animal [44]. In tumour-bearing or tumour-immunised hosts anti-tumour Ab are frequently found. These Ab also recognise proteins in normal tissue and hence are not tumour specific. It is an enigma as to whether the Ab response is to be considered a true anti-tumour response or rather reflects the breaking of tolerance to normal, e.g. differentiation antigens. T lymphocytes play a key, if not the most important, role in tumour immunity. In contrast to the serological definition of antigens by a variety of techniques such as immunoprecipitation, Western blotting and others, it has been difficult to structurally analyse T-cell defined antigens on tumour cells. The difficulty lies in the fact that TCR are expressed in the membrane of the T lymphocyte, and that the response against the TAA is MHC restricted. Therefore, only a few T-cell defined tumour antigens have now been characterised in some detail in experimental animal model systems. However, characterisation of T cell defined human tumour antigens by biochemical techniques is developing [45, 46]. This technique involves the stimulation of T lymphocytes by proteins which have been isolated by biochemical separation, together with antigen presenting cells (APC). Mucins of pancreatic, breast and colon tumours are the human TAA best characterised so far [47]. These mucins have a characteristic polyvalent structure and are able to stimulate CTL in an MHC-unrestricted fashion, but do involve the TCR$\alpha\beta$ [48, 49]. Such mucins are also expressed in normal epithelium and this raises the question as to the basis of specificity of the immune response to mucins. Why this does not result in the in vivo elimination of tumour cells is still a major question, but it might be due to the relative lack of functional CD4$^+$ T helper cells. Further studies at the structural and cellular levels may provide the tools necessary to boost the human anti-mucinous cancer response.

In brief, rather than tumour-specific molecules, cancer cells express tumour-specific epitopes of common molecules. Therefore, the original idea that tumour antigens are lineage-specific differentiation antigens deserves renewed attention. This is even more so in view of our advanced understanding of antigen presentation by MHC-class-I antigens, which point in the direction that any modification in a coding gene can, in principle, be recognised by the cellular immune system. The fact that CTL defined antigens are shared by human tumours of different histologic origin [50, 51] or MHC-class-I HLA-A2 matched allogenic melanoma cells indeed illustrates that common genetic alterations accompany malignant transformation. In the latter case it has been speculated, that melanoma cells carry common melanoma TAA, that are recognised by CTL in a MHC-class-I restricted fashion.

5. IL-2 and cancer

The unique specificity of the immune response provided the field with its own language and mechanisms. With the discovery and characterisation of the working mechanisms of various lymphokines, it has become clear that many of these molecules obey the same rules of interaction as followed by classic hormones and their receptors. Under physiological conditions lymphokines represent short range signalling molecules between immune cells characterised by short half life and transient expression. Many interleukins have now been identified, but no detailed knowledge of their mode of action is yet present. IL-2 is one of the most extensively studied lymphokines and its pivotal role for the generation of an effective immune response has been well established. IL-2 is critical as well as sufficient for the expansion of most immature and mature T cells, NK cells and B cells during various phases of their immune response. It is involved in intrathymic T-cell maturation and differentiation [52], the in vivo development of virus-specific CTL [53], and the expansion of NK lymphocytes [54] as well as maintenance of antigen specific T lymphocytes [55]. IL-2 promotes and maintains long term in vitro expansion of activated T cells [9, 56] and as such, it represents a key biological response modifier (BRM) for the activation of immune lymphocytes. IL-2 also plays a central role in the communication between the two major populations of the immune system: the T and B lymphocytes. Like many other interleukins, IL-2 exerts different tasks in the immune network, all with common characteristics, e.g., the triggering of their production is rapid, their range of action and half lives are short and they modulate the behaviour of multiple different cell types: pleiotropic activity. IL-2 does not only activate cells and allow them to proliferate but also effect adhesion molecules in multiple ways. Interleukins effect cell adhesion receptors, which themselves can act like lymphokine receptors to receptors for lymphokines that can promote cell-to-cell adhesion, and the adhesion in turn determines the response of cells to cytokines [57]. Therefore, the administration of IL-2 and other lymphokines does not only effect individual cells of the immune system, but also acts on other tissues in the body thereby affecting the homing patterns of immune lymphocytes among other cell types. It may become clear from the contributions elsewhere in this book that IL-2 allows the design of powerful immunotherapeutic strategies. This wide range of IL-2 driven activities makes this cytokine a powerful tool in immunotherapy. It can now be produced in quantity by recombinant DNA-technology.

Because of the complexities of IL-2 actions on distinct immune cells and other tissues immunotherapy with cytokines can be considered to be in its infancy. Usually, lymphokines are applied systematically and, due to their short half life in vivo, the therapeutic effect requires high doses causing severe toxic side-effects. This is well documented for IL-2. From the clinical trials performed so far it is clear that treatment with IL-2 alone and IL-2 plus autologous IL-2 activated lymphocytes has been shown to cause tumour regression in patients with metastatic melanoma or renal cell cancer [58]. The investigation of the clinical effect of IL-2 involved in the regulation of immune recognition and immunologic effector mechanisms is difficult. No simple laboratory tests have revealed correlations with tumour responses. The in vitro tests available today do not predict the physiological or clinical impact of a given lymphokine treatment and underscore the urgency of designing in vitro tests, which are relevant for the monitoring of immunotherapy in general. A major goal of IL-2 treatment has been the increase of MHC-unrestricted or so-called non-specific immune resistance to cancer. Future strategies for the treatment of human cancer will involve transduction of IL-2 (and other lymphokine) genes into tumour cells and subsequent reinfusion of these genetically manipulated cells at the tumour site which induce an immune-inflammatory reaction. This reaction may then provoke MHC-unrestricted as well as MHC-restricted lymphocyte anti-tumour responses. Such studies will eventually show whether tumour-restricted immunogenicity against human tumours can be obtained as the relevant endpoint [59].

6. Immune network and tumour cell escape from immune attack

From the immune principles and mechanisms described above it can be summarised that, depending on the type and strength of activation stimulus delivered to lymphocytes, which in the case of tumour cells is dictated by the nature of the TAA and how these TAA are presented on the tumour cell surface, a cascade of immune regulatory events follows. This involves modulation of the expression of TCR or putative NK cell receptor, of cytokine receptors, of lymphocyte cell surface adhesion/signal-transducing molecules. Induction of distinct lymphokine repertoires also takes place. In turn, these events result in the activation of other T and B cell subsets, their proliferation and differentiation into effector cells. Each of these cells is capable of producing their own lymphokine repertoire. Eventually the elimination of tumour cells may follow. This enormous complexity of interaction reflects the fine regulatory mechanisms of the immune system to combat foreign invaders, including cancer cells [for review 4, 5].

One may then ask: why do tumour cells arise in vivo, in spite of a functioning immune system as we also find it in cancer patients? The answer lies in the ability of tumour cells to generate escape mechanisms. Cancer cells are known to produce their own cytokines such as prostaglandins or transforming growth factors (TGFs). A number of these cytokines antagonise the immune response against tumours thereby protecting the cancer cells against the immune attack. Moreover, cancer cells may show aberrant MHC expression and hence, even when tumour-specific antigens or TAA are expressed, these may not be adequately presented to the immune system.

Furthermore, tumour cells of particular histogenetic origin have also been shown to lack the expression of costimulatory ligands such as ICAM-1, and these integrin-LFA interactions were shown to be critical for the differentiation of lymphocytes into effector cells [36]. The therapeutic administration of IL-2 can override these immune suppressive functions of tumour cells and their cytokines on the one hand, and, at the same time promote lymphocyte proliferation and antitumour effector functions of immune cells.

7. Immunotherapy of cancer

7.1. Introduction

The state of art using IL-2 alone or in combination with other cytokines and/or with lymphokine activated lymphocytes is discussed here and in detail elsewhere in this issue. It suffices to say that although clear therapeutic anti-tumour effects have been obtained, they are as yet unsatisfactory.

Therefore, we have focused on new strategies for circumventing the difficulties in generating T-cell specific anti-tumour responses due to either lack of immunogenic TAA or due to the lack of costimulatory ligands on the

tumour cells. We combine:
a. the tumour selectivity of mAb,
b. the cytolytic capacity of in vitro activated and expanded T cells and
c. the immune proliferation and T-cell activity enhancing capacity of IL-2 for immunotherapy.

7.2. Bispecific monoclonal antibody (bs-mAb) triggered lysis of tumour cells by CTL

An increasing number of mAb have now been well characterised and which are capable of selectively binding to human tumour cells or to lymphocyte cell surface activation molecules. Somatic hybridisation of two myeloma clones, each secreting a mAb with the desired specificity, i.e. recognising CTL activation sites on the one hand and TAA on the tumour cell on the other, produces a quadroma, which now secretes a mAb with dual specificity. One Ab binding site recognising the TAA and the other the CTL, for instance, the CD3 activation molecule of the TCR complex [60]. Because of their dual specificity these bs-mAb also facilitate the bridging of the cytotoxic T cell to the TAA expressing tumour cell. The bridging of the T cell to the tumour cell by the bs-mAb now results in activation of the CTL which, in turn, causes the delivery of a lethal hit to that tumour cell. Moreover, it also triggers the production of lymphokines by these CTL (Figure 3). This novel approach circumvents the need to isolate T cells with tumour specificity, which has proven to be so difficult (see above). The binding of the CTL to the tumour cell is now mediated by the bs-mAb and there is, therefore, no need for the expression of MHC on the tumour cells which is normally required for the triggering of CTL.

IL-2 is essential for the in vitro large scale expansion of the patients' own lymphocytes required for this form of therapy. The combined use of in vitro activated and expanded CTL and tumour-selective bs-mAb has been shown to be an efficient effector mechanism for the lysis of tumour cells in mice and man [61–66]. The in vivo administration of IL-2 together with the IL-2 activated and expanded lymphocytes, pre-targeted with the bs-mAb, will promote T-lymphocyte viability and anti-tumour activity. The potential of this approach is impressive. Indeed, mAb with specificity for particular lymphocyte activation sites exist, that is, NK cells, $\alpha\beta$ or $\gamma\delta$ TCR expressing T cells. Each mAb triggers different functions or lymphocyte subpopulations. Their selective use thus allows the activation and expansion of particular subsets of lymphocytes without the need for prior isolation of these lymphocyte subsets. Humanisation of the mouse bs-mAb will lower their in vivo antigenicity and reduce the human anti-mouse Ab response, which interferes with their action.

We and others have started a phase I–II clinical trial employing such bs-mAb retargeted lymphocytes for the intraperitoneal treatment of ovarian cancer patients (see below) [67].

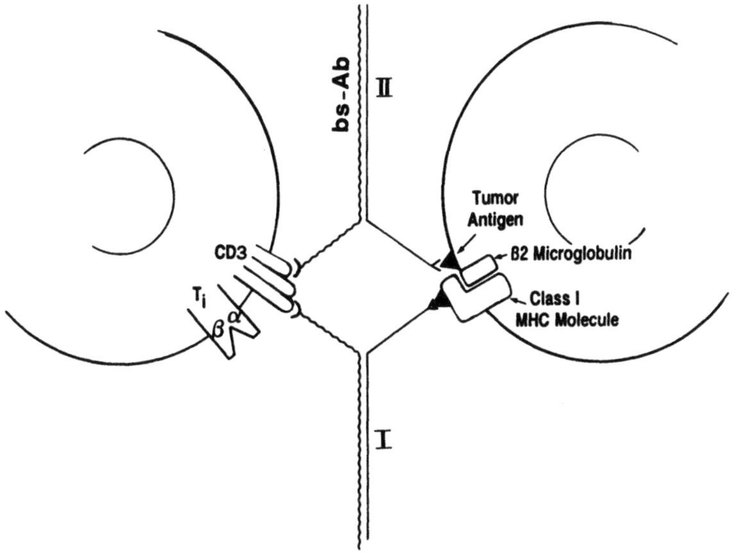

Figure 3. Bispecific Antibody triggered cytolysis of CD8 following targeting of the CTL to the target cell.

7.3. Construction of chimeric Ig/TCR expressing T cells

Another way of endowing T lymphocytes with an Ig-dictated antigen specificity is to construct chimeric Ig/TCR genes that can be transfected to T lymphocytes, resulting in the functional expression of such chimeric receptors on their surface. In model systems it has recently been shown that such genetically engineered lymphocytes functionally express the chimeric Ig/TCR receptors, resulting in the activation of lymphokine production and triggering of the lytic machinery following binding to TAA on cancer cells [68]. There are a number of reasons for developing this technology for clinical use:

1. bs-mAb targeted T lymphocytes retain the Ab-dictated specificity only for limited periods of time (6–72 h), due to the dissociation of the bs-mAb from the surface [57; Bolhuis, manuscript in preparation];
2. T lymphocytes expressing the chimeric Ig/TCR may show normal migration and homing capacities.

Consequently, bs-mAb targeted T lymphocytes may then be most effective when applied locoregionally, whereas the chimeric Ig/TCR expressing lymphocytes can also be administered systematically. Another advantage is that Ig/TCR expressing T lymphocytes may show T cell memory function. If so they can provide the patient with a long lasting protective immunity against the tumour cells. Before clinical application of these genetically modified lymphocytes is effected we have to know whether the administration of these lymphocytes is safe. Theoretically their genetic manipulation might initiate an oncogenic transformation. The results obtained in vitro, and in laboratory animals, and those obtained during and after 60 months of observation of patients, who received neogene transfected autologous T lymphocytes, have not, however, revealed any abnormalities or side effects.

8. Clinical results

8.1. The treatment of ovarian cancer with Bs-mab CTL and IL-2

Most of the patients with ovarian cancer have tumour outside the small pelvis (FIGO stage III) at the time of diagnosis. The tumour dissemination is usually restricted to the abdomen, even in advanced disease, which makes these patients good candidates for intraperitoneal (i.p.) treatment. Intravenous (i.v.) administration of a platinum analog and an alkylating agent is the standard treatment for advanced ovarian cancer resulting in a response rate of 70–80%. The 5-year survival rates are, however, only 20–30% due to frequent relapse. The median survival time from the start of induction of second-line chemotherapy is less than one year [69] and this calls for the design of novel treatment modalities. This prompted us to start a phase II study, using a bs-mAb, called OC-TR, of which one F(ab') binding site is directed against the CD3 activation site on the CTL and the other against an ovarian TAA (MOv18) [70]. The parental MOv18 mAb, conjugated with fluorescing isothiocyanate, showed positive staining of 100% of the mucinous carcinoma frozen ovarian cancer sections, and almost all cells of the sections stained positive. The selectivity of MOv18 mAb was demonstrated by its lack of cross reactivity, i.e., only 3 of 141 sections (only 2% of non-ovarian tumour sections stained positive). Normal tissues from kidneys, spleen, bladder, ovary, uterus, prostate, pancreas, colon, stomach, liver, skin, parotid gland, thyroid, larynx, breast, testis, lung, bone marrow and peripheral blood lymphocytes did not bind the MOv18 mAb. The OC-TR bs-mAb induces 80 percent lysis of ovarian carcinoma cells in a 4-hour 51-Cr release assay at an effector CTL to target cell ratio of 30:1 [65, 70, 71]. In a clinical study using 131-iodine labelled MOv-18 in 18 ovarian cancer patients positive images were obtained in 27 of 32 lesions detected at laparotomy [72].

We have used bs-mAb (OC-TR) targeted CTL with IL-2 for the treatment of ovarian cancer patients who relapsed after first-line chemotherapy. Prior to treatment tumour biopsies were obtained during laparoscopy and examined for the presence of the MOv18 relevant TAA. When the biopsy of the patient showed reactivity with the MOv18 mAb the patient proceeded to a debulking laparotomy, at which time the remaining measurable and valuable indicator lesions were documented. A Tenckhoff catheter was then inserted. One day before surgery about 30ml of blood is drawn from the patient and the isolated lymphoid cells are cultured and activated with IL-2 and phytohemagglutinin (PHA) to induce cell proliferation. After about 2–3 weeks of in vitro culture a 50-fold proliferation of lymphocytes has taken place. The majority of the expanded lymphocyte population is $CD3^+$. The in vitro expanded lymphocytes are then targeted with OC-TR and tested in the laboratory for their cytolytic capacity. These OC-TR targeted and activated lymphocytes are infused ip in 500ml saline with 600,000 IU of IL-2 at numbers of 10^9 lymphocytes per day, for 5 days, via the Tenckhoff catheter. After 3 weeks this treatment cycle is repeated. Eight weeks after the last infusion of OC-TR targeted CTL + IL-2 the response is evaluated during laparotomy.

Eight patients are presently on study and 6 have completed therapy. Fever and anorexia were the most prominent side effects and could be easily managed. Three patients, who had tumour positive ascites became negative within 5 days of therapy. The ascites became infiltrated with lymphocytes, eosinophils and granulocytes. In 2 out of 3 valuable patients one partial and one complete regression of tumour was observed. In one of these patients retroperitoneal lymph node metastases had progressed, in the other new submucosal bowel metastases were seen.

Taken together, these data suggest that the regression of the intraperitoneal tumour was due to the immunotherapy. The other patients treated showed extraperitoneal metastasis and therefore no explorative laparotomy was done rendering these patients invaluable. The preliminary results suggest that the anticipated inflammatory immune response is indeed evoked and with effective antitumour activity, but that systematic immunity against the tumours may not be generated effectively.

8.2. The treatment of renal cancer with IL-2 and α-interferon (α-IFN)

With the use of a combination of IL-2 and α-IFN, encouraging results have been obtained in cancer treatment [73, 74]. We have begun a study of IL-2 with α-IFN and IL-2 activated lymphocytes (LAK). Patients entered into this phase II study had undergone nephrectomy. The treatment schedule is presented in Table 1. Thirty one patients have now been entered and 28 can be evaluated for response; two are too early, one is lost to follow-up. The median age of the patients was 54 years (30-70), median performance status (WHO) was 0. Two patients had previously received radiotherapy. Metastasis were present in all patients: seventeen patients showed 2 or more metastatic organ sites. Three patients showed a CR (11%), and PR was observed in a further ten patients (36%). The duration of the CR response is $8–21^+$ months, and of the PR response 3–17 months. The median survival of the treated patients exceeds 24 months. The high overall response rate of 47% observed so far compares favourably with the results reported for IL-2 alone [75–77] or IL-2 in combination with LAK [75, 76, 78, 79].

Table 1. Induction and maintenance treatment scheme of IL2 with LAK and aIFN in metastatic renal cell cancer.

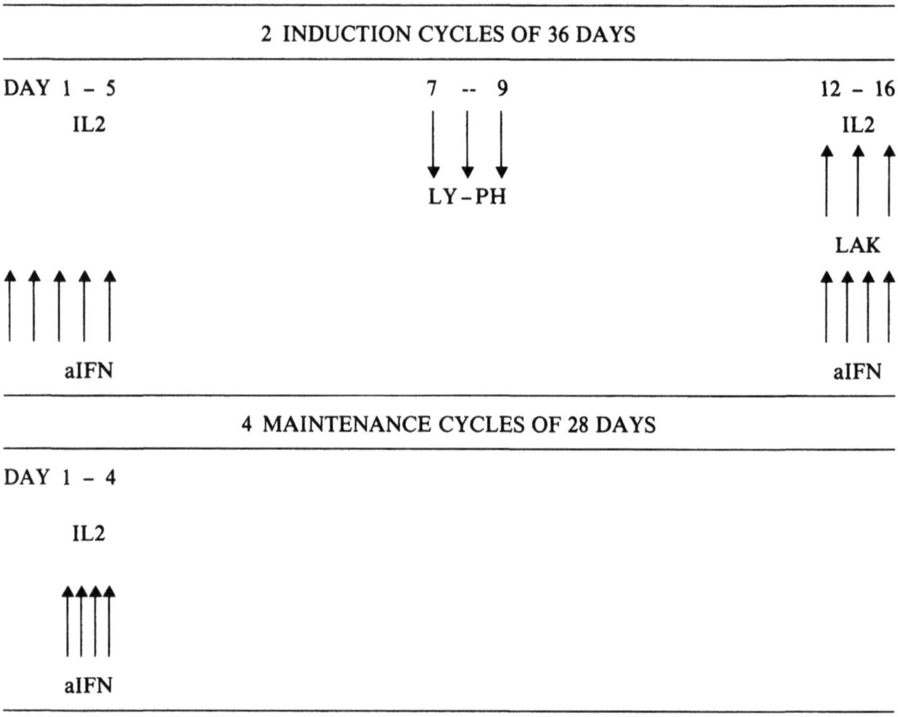

IL2 18 MIU/m²/day CIV; aIFN 4MU/m²/day IM
LY-PH = lympho-pheresis

9. Perspectives: questions to be addressed

The clinical applications that become feasible by using the targeting of immune lymphocytes to tumour cells by either bs-mAb or by their chimeric Ig/TCR are evident. To select for the most optimal procedure we have to know whether the triggering of cytolysis by the CTL is important or rather that the induction of lymphokine production by particular subsets of lymphocytes, including non-CTL, is the more critical factor. Moreover, depending on the localisation of the tumour various subsets of the lymphocytes may be required for immunotherapy, because the distinct subsets have particular trafficking and homing capacities. We also need to prepare batches of bs-mAb and lymphocytes expressing chimeric Ig/TCR with specificities for distinct epitopes on the same TAA or for different TAA on the tumour in order to circumvent heterogeneity in the expression of TAA on cancer cells.

Many investigators are currently addressing these questions. This should, however, not delay the clinical application of these principles, because the reagents and technologies are already at hand. Only their clinical in vivo application will provide the relevant data to allow the further refinement of these immunotherapeutic strategies.

References

1. Ehrlich P. Uber den Jetzigen Stand der Karzinomforschung. Ned Tijdschr Geneeskd 1909; 35: 273–90.
2. Burnet FM. The concept of immunological surveillance. Progr Exper Tumor Res 1970; 13: 1–27.
3. Lloyd KO, Old LJ. Human monoclonal antibodies to glycolipids and other carbohydrate antigens. Dissection of the humoral immune response in cancer patients. Cancer Res 1989; 49: 3445–51.
4. Hersey P, Bolhuis RLH. Non-specific MHC-unrestricted killer cells and their receptors. Immunol Today 1987; 8: 233–9.
5. Bolhuis RLHB, Braakman E. Lymphocyte-mediated responses: activation of, and lysis by, cytotoxic lymphocytes. Curr Opin Immunol 1988; 1: 236–40.
6. Köhler G, Milstein C. Continuous cultures of fused cells secreting antibody of predefined specificity. Nature 1975; 256: 495–7.
7. Acuto O, Hussey RE, Fitzgerald KA, et al. The human T-cell receptor: Appearance in ontogeny and biochemical relationship of α and β subunits on IL-2 dependent clones and T-cell tumors. Cell 1983; 34: 717–26.
8. Staertz UD, Pasternack MS, Klein JR, et al. Monoclonal antibodies specific for a murine cytotoxic T-lymphocyte clone. Proc Natl Acad Sci USA 1984; 1799–803.
9. Bolhuis RLH, Gravekamp C, Van de Griend RJ. Cell-Cell interactions. Clin Immunol Allergy 1986; 6: 29–90.
10. Lanier L, Ruitenberg JJ, Phillips JH. Human $CD3^+$ T lymphocytes that express neither CD4 nor CD8. J Exp Med 1986; 164: 339–44.
11. Ferrini SG, Bottino C, Blassoni R, et al. Characterization of $CD3^+$, $CD4^-$, $CD8^-$ clones expressing the putative T-cell receptor gamma gene product. J Exp Med 1987; 166: 277–82.
12. Borst J, Van de Griend R, Van Oostveen H, et al. A T-cell receptor γ/CD3 complex found on cloned functional lymphocytes. Nature 1987; 325: 683–8.
13. Brenner MB, McLean J, Scheft H, et al. Two forms of the T-cell receptor gamma protein found on peripheral blood cytotoxic T lymphocytes. Nature 1987; 325: 689–94.
14. Van de Griend RJ, Tax WJM, Van Krimpen BA, et al. Lysis of tumor cells by $CD3^+$, 4^-, 8^-, 16^+ T-cell receptor $\alpha\beta^-$-clones regulated via CD3 and CD16 activation sites, recombinant interleukin 2 and interferon β. J Immunol 1987; 138: 1627–33.
15. Sturm E, Braakman E, Bontrop RE, et al. Coordinated Vγ and Vδ gene-segment rearrangements in human T-cell receptor γ/δ^+ lymphocytes. Eur J Immunol 1989; 19: 1261–5.
16. Bluestone JA, Crom RQ, Cotterman M, et al. Structure and specificty of T-cell receptor $\gamma\delta$ on major histocompatibility complex antigen specific $CD3^+$, $CD4^-$, $CD8^-$ T lymphocytes. J Exp Med 1988; 168: 1899–916.
17. Haregewoin A, Soman G, Hom RC, Finberg RW. Human $\gamma\delta^+$ T cells respond to mycobacterial heat-shock protein. Nature 1989; 340: 309–12.
18. Paliard X, Yssel H, Blanchard D, et al. Antigen specific and MHC non-restricted cytotoxicity of T cell receptor $\alpha\beta^+$ and $\gamma\delta^+$ human T-cell clones isolated in IL-4. J Immunol 1989; 143: 452–7.
19. Kozbor D, Trinchieri G, Monos DS, et al. Human TCR-γ^+/δ^+, $CD8^+$ T lymphocytes recognize tetanus toxoid in a MHC restricted fashion. J Exp Med 1989; 169: 1847–51.
20. Holoshitz J, Koning F, Coligan JE, et al. Isolation of $CD4^-$, $CD8^-$ mycobacteria-reactive T lymphocyte clones from rheumatoid arthrites synovial fluid. Nature 1989; 339: 226–9.

21. Sturm E, Braakman E, Fisch P, et al. Human Vγ9-Vδ2 TCRγδ lymphocytes show specificity to Daudi Burkitt's lymphoma cells. J Immunol 1990; 145: 3202–8.
22. Fisch P, Malkovsky M, Braakman E, et al. Gamma/delta T cell clones and natural killer cell clones mediate distinct cytolysis. J Exp Med 1990; 171: 1567–79.
23. Davis MM, Bjorkman PJ. T-cell antigen receptor genes and T-cell recognition. Nature 1988; 334: 395–402.
24. Trinchieri G. Biology of Natural Killer Cells. In: Advances in Immunology. New York: Academic Press, 1989; 187–376.
25. Seeley JK, Golub SH. Studies on cytotoxity generated in human mixed lymphocyte cultures: 1. Time Course and Target spectrum of Several Distinct Concomitant Cytotoxic Activities. J Immunol 1978; 120: 1415–22.
26. Poros A, Klein E. Distinction of Anti-K562 and Anti-Allocytotoxity in in vitro Stimulated Populations of Human Lymphocytes. Cell Immunol 1979; 46: 57–68.
27. Masucci MG, Klein E, Argrov S. Disappearance of the NK effect after explantation of lymphocytes and generation of similar nonspecific cytotoxity correlated to the level of blastogenesis in activated cultures. J Immunol 1980; 124: 2458–63.
28. Hersey P, Bindon C, Edwards A. Induction of cytotoxic activity in human lymphocytes against autologous and allogeneic melanoma cells in vitro by culture with interleukin 2. Int J Cancer 1981; 28: 695–703.
29. Vose BM, Bonnard GD. Specific cytotoxicity against autologous tumour and proliferative responses of human lymphocytes grown in interleukin 2. Int J Cancer 1982; 29: 33–9.
30. Grimm EA, Mazumder A, Zhang HZ, Rosenberg SA. Lymphokine-activated killer cells phenomenon or lysis of natural killer-resistant fresh solid tumor cells by Interleukin 2-activated autologous human peripheral blood lymphocytes. J Exp Med 1982; 155: 1823–41.
31. Bolhuis RLH, Ronteltap CPM. Generation of natural killer (NK) cell activity after mixed lymphocyte culture (MLC): activation of effector cells in NK cell-depleted cell populations. Immunol Lett 1980; 1: 191–6.
32. Bolhuis RLH, Schellekens SH. Induction of natural killer cell activity and allocytotoxicity in human peripheral blood lymphocytes after mixed lymphocyte culture. Scand J Immunol 1981; 13: 401–12.
33. Van de Griend RJ, Giphart MJ, Van Krimpen BA, Bolhuis RLH. Human T-cell clones exerting multiple cytolytic activities show heterogeneity in susceptibility to inhibition by monoclonal antibodies. J Immunol 1984; 133: 1222–9.
34. Clevers H, Alarcon B, Wileman T, Terhorst C. The T Cell Receptor/CD3 Complex: A Dynamic Protein Ensemble. Annu Rev Immunol 1988; 6: 629–62.
35. Geppert TD, Davis LS, Gur H, et al. Accessory Cell Signals Involved in T-cell Activation. Immunol Rev 1990; 117: 1–66.
36. Goedegebuure SP, Segal DM, Braakman E, et al. Induction of lysis by TCR $\gamma\delta^{+}$/$CD3^{+}$ T lymphocytes via CD2 requires triggering via the T11,1 epitope only. J Immunol 1989; 142: 1797–802.
37. Braakman E, Goedegebuure PS, Vreugdenhil RJ, et al. ICAM melanoma cells are relatively resistant to CD3 mediated T-cell lysis. Int J Cancer 1990; 46: 475–80.
38. Pantaleo G, Olive D, Poggi A, et al. Antibody-induced modulation of the CD3/T-cell receptor complex causes T-cell refractoriness by inhibiting the early metabolic steps involved in T-cell activation. J Exp Med 1987; 166: 619–24.
39. Bolhuis RLH, Roozemond RC, Van de Griend RJ. Induction and blocking of cytolysis in $CD2^{+}$ $CD3^{-}$ NK and $CD2^{+}$ $CD3^{+}$ cytotoxic T lymphocytes via CD2 50-Kd sheep erythrocyte receptor. J Immunol 1986; 136: 3939–44.
40. Moingeon P, Chang HC, Wallner BP, et al. CD2-mediated adhesion facilitates T-Lymphocyte antigen recognition function. Nature 1989; 339: 312–4.
41. Van Seventer GA, Shimizu Y, Shaw S. Roles of multiple accessory molecules in T-cell activation. Curr Opin Immunol 1991; 3: 294–303.
42. Shimizu Y, Shaw S. Lymphocyte interactions with extracellular matrix. Faseb J 1991; 5: 2292–9.

43. Old LJ, Boyse EA. Antigens of tumors and leukemias induced by viruses. Proc Fed 1965; 24: 1009–17.
44. Srivastava PK, Old LJ. Individually distinct transplantation antigen of chemically induced mouse tumors. Immunol Today 1988; 9: 78–83.
45. Hersey P, Meldrum C, Daniels V, et al. Characterization of melanoma antigens recognized by human T cells. In: Finn OJ, Lotze M, editors. Cellular immunity and the immunotherapy of cancer. New York: Wiley-Liss, 1990: 343–9.
46. Notter M, Schirrmacher V. Tumor specific T cell clones recognize different protein determinants of autologous human melanoma cells. Int J Cancer 1990; 45: 834–41.
47. Gendler S, Taylor-Papadimitriou J, Duhlig T, et al. A highly immunogenic region of a human polymorphic epithelial mucin expressed by carcinomas is made up of tandem repeats. J Biol Chem 1988; 263: 12820–3.
48. Barnd DL, Lan M, Metzgar R, Finn OJ. Specific, MHC-unrestricted recognition of tumor-associated mucins by human cytotoxic T cells. Proc Natl Acad Sci USA 1989; 86: 7159–63.
49. Jerome KR, Barnd DL, Bendt KM, et al. Cytotoxic T lymphocytes derived from patients with breast adenocarcinoma recognize an epitope present on the protein core of a mucin molecule preferentially expressed by malignant cells. Cancer Res 1991; 51: 2908–16.
50. Slovin SF, Lackman RD, Ferrone S, et al. Cellular immune response to human sarcomas: Cytotoxic T cell clones reactive with autologous sarcomas. I. Development, phenotype and specificity. J Immunol 1986; 137: 3042–8.
51. Crowley NJ, Slingluff CL, Darrow TL, Seigler HF. Generation of human autologous melanoma-specific cytotoxic T-cells using HLA-A2-matched allogeneic melanomas. Cancer Res 1990; 50: 492–8.
52. Tentori L, Longo DL, Zuniga-Pflucker JC, et al. Essential role of the interleukin-2-receptor pathways in thymocyte maturation in vivo. J Exp Med 1988; 168: 1741–8.
53. Leist TP, Kohler M, Eppler M, Zinkernagel RM. Effects of treatment with IL-2 receptor specific monoclonal antibody in mice: inhibition of cytotoxic T cell responses but not of T help. J Immunol 1989; 143: 628–32.
54. Biron CA, Young HA, Kasauan MT. Interleukin-2-induced proliferation of murine natural killer cells in vivo. J Exp Med 1990; 171: 173–88.
55. Chen W, Reese VA, Cheever MA. Adoptively transferred antigen-specific T cells can be grown and maintained in large numbers in vivo for extended periods of time by intermittent restimulation with specific antigen plus IL-2. J Immunol 1990; 144: 3659–66.
56. Van de Griend RJ, Ronteltap CPM, Gravekamp C, et al. Interferon β and recombinant IL-2 can both enhance but by different pathways, the non-specific cytolytic potential of $T3^-$ natural killer cell derived clones rather than that of $T3^+$ clones. J Immunol 1986; 5: 1700–7.
57. Oettgen HF, Old LJ. The history of cancer immunotherapy. In: DeVita VT, Hellman S, Rosenberg SA, editors. Biologic therapy of cancer. Philadelphia: Lippincott, 1991: 87–199.
58. Nathan C, Sporn M. Cytokines in context. J Cell Biol 1991; 981–6.
59. Rosenberg SA, Lotze MT, Muul LM, et al. Observations on the systemic administration of autologous lymohokine-activated killer cells and recombinant interleukin-2 to patients with metastatic cancer. N Engl J Med 1985; 313: 1485–92.
60. Milstein C, Cuello AC. Hybrid hybridomas and their use in immunohistochemistry. Nature 1983; 305: 537–40.
61. Lanzavecchia A, Scheidegger D. The use of hybrid hybridomas to target human cytotoxic T lymphocytes. Eur J Immunol 1987; 17: 105–11.
62. Titus JA, Garrido MA, Hecht TT, et al. Human T cells targeted with anti-T3 cross-linked to antitumor antibody prevent tumor growth in nude mice. J Immunol 1987; 138: 4018–22.
63. Canevari S, Ménard S, Mezzanzanica D, et al. Anti-ovarian carcinoma anti-T3 heteroconjugates or hybrid antibodies induce tumor cell lysis by cytotoxic T-cells. Int J Cancer 1988; Suppl. 2: 18–21.
64. Van Dijk J, Tsuruo T, Segal DM, et al. Bispecific antibodies reactive with the multidrug-resistance-related glycoprotein and CD3 induce lysis of multidrug-resistant tumor cells. Int J

Cancer 1989; 44: 738–43.
65. Van Dijk J, Warnaar SO, Van Eendenburg JDH, et al. Induction of Tumor-cell lysis by bi-specific monoclonal antibodies recognizing renal-cell carcinoma and CD3 antigen. Int J Cancer 1989; 43: 344–9.
66. Van de Griend RJ, Bolhuis RLH, Stoter G, Roozemond RC. Regulation of cytolytic activity in $CD3^-$ and $CD3^+$ killer cell clones by monoclonal antibodies (anti-CD16, anti-CD2, anti-CD3) depends on subclass specificity of target cell IgG-FcR. J Immunol 1987; 138: 3137–44.
67. Nitta T, Sato K, Yagita H, et al. Preliminary trial of specific targeting therapy against malignant glioma. Lancet 1990; 335: 368–71.
68. Gross G, Waks T, Eshhar Z. Expression of immunoglobulin-T-cell receptor chimeric molecules as functional receptors with antibody-type specificity. Proc Natl Acad Sci USA 1989; 86: 10024–8.
69. Burg van der MEL, Hoff AM, Lent van M, et al. Carboplatin and cyclophosphamide salvage therapy for ovarian cancer patients relapsing after cisplatin combination chemotherapy. Eur J Cancer 1991; 27: 248–50.
70. Mezzanzanica D, Canevari S, Ménard S, et al. Human ovarian carcinoma lysis by cytotoxic T cells targeted by bispecific monoclonal antibodies: analysis of the antibody components. Int J Cancer 1988; 41: 609–15.
71. Pupa SM, Canevari S, Fontanelli R, et al. Activation of mononuclear cells to be used for hybrid monoclonal antibody-induced lysis of human ovarian carcinoma cells. Int J Cancer 1988; 42: 455–9.
72. Colnaghi MI, Buraggi GL, Canevari S, et al. Evaluation of the suitability of a monoclonal antibody raised against human ovarian carcinoma for therapeutic approaches. Nucl Med Biol 1989; 16: 633–6.
73. Cameron RB, McIntosh JK, Rosenberg SA. Synergistic antitumor effects of combination immunotherapy with recombinant hybrid alpha-interferon in the treatment of established murine hepatic metastases. Cancer Res 1988; 48: 5810–7.
74. Rosenberg SA, Schwartz S, Spiess PJ. Combination immunotherapy for cancer: synergistic antitumor interactions of interleukin-2, alpha-interferon, and tumor-infiltrating lymphocytes. J Natl Cancer Inst 1988; 80: 1393–7.
75. Negrier S, Philip T, Stoter G, et al. Interleukin-2 with or without LAK cells in metastatic renal cell carcinoma: A report of a European multicentre study. Eur J Cancer Clin Oncol 1989; 25: S21–S8.
76. Rosenberg SA, Lotze MT, Yang JC, et al. Experience with the use of high-dose interleukin-2 in the treatment of 652 cancer patients. Ann Surg 1989; 210: 474–85.
77. Abrams JS, Rayner AA, Wiernik PH, et al. High-dose recombinant interleukin-2 alone: A regimen with limited activity in the treatment of advanced renal cell carcinoma. J Natl Cancer Inst 1990; 82: 1202–6.
78. Fisher RI, Coltman CA, Doroshow JH, et al. Metastatic renal cancer treated with interleukin-2 and lymphokine-activated killer cells. Ann Int Med 1988; 108: 518–23.
79. Parkinson DR, Fisher RI, Rayner AA, et al. Therapy of renal cell carcinoma with interleukin-2 and lymphokine-activated killer cells: Phase II experience with a hybrid bolus and continuous infusion interleukin-2 regimen. J Clin Oncol 1990; 8: 1630–6.

9. Interleukin-2 and other cytokines

JENS ATZPODIEN, AXEL SCHOMBURG, HARTMUT KIRCHNER,
and HUBERT POLIWODA

In combining recombinant human interleukin-2 (IL-2) with other cytokines, a plethora of immunologic effects are exploited. Most of these host defense mechanisms, effects on tumour growth and on tumour differentiation are not yet fully understood [72].

Interleukin-2 is believed to exert its anti-tumour potential via the cellular and humoral activation of a broad spectrum of immune functions [5]. Among these multiple IL-2 mediated effects in vivo there is evidence for a non-linear dose response curve i.e., 'optimal' biologic response has been observed far below the maximum cytokine dose used and/or tolerated in man [143, 154].

Previously, employing IL-2 for the induction of high affinity (i.e., alpha and beta chain) binding sites we found that increased proportions of human peripheral blood mononuclear cells would respond to IL-2 in vitro upon dose reduction from 1,000 to 1 international unit (IU) per ml of cell culture (Figure 1). This initial observation was confirmed in a phase I dose escalation trial in patients with advanced malignancy; upon subcutaneous (SC) administration of IL-2, we found a non-linear induction of the alpha chain IL-2 receptor. Thus, single doses of 1.8 million IU per m^2 i.e., ten to thirty-fold below the maximum tolerated dose of IL-2 in human, produced IL-2 receptor positivity of circulating lymphocytes at 'maximum' levels which were not increased by further dose escalation (Figure 2A).

While both pre-clinical and clinical models support the concept of a non-linear dose response curve for IL-2 (Table 1), this is not pertinent to all immunologic functions mediated by this cytokine. Rather, it is believed that various biologic activities of IL-2 follow different dose response correlations. In an attempt to characterize the IL-2 driven expansion of circulating natural killer (NK) cells i.e., CD56 positive lymphocytes in vivo, we observed a dose-dependent and almost linear induction of NK cells over a 'therapeutic' range of SC IL-2 from 1.8 to 14.4 million IU per m^2 per dose (Figure 2B).

While IL-2 as single agent is known to mediate a wide array of different biologic actions, it is conceivable that the preclinical and clinical use of IL-2 in combination with other cytokines opens up an even broader spectrum of immunomodulatory functions.

J. Wagstaff (ed.), The Role of Interleukin-2 in the Treatment of Cancer Patients, 141-167.

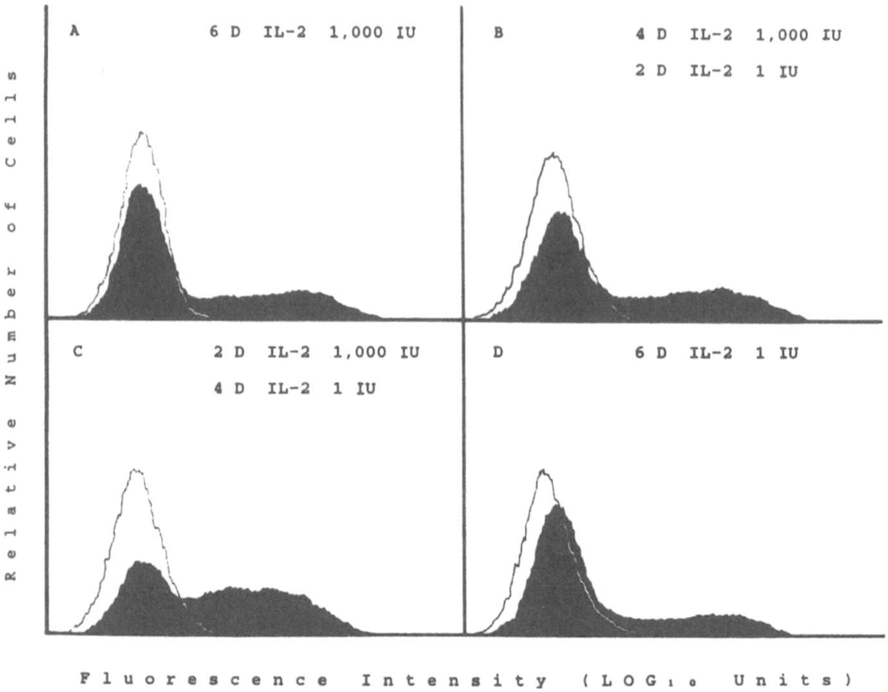

Figure 1. Effects of various concentrations of IL-2 on the expression of alpha chain IL-2 receptors by human peripheral blood mononuclear cells (PBMC) in vitro.
Over a 6-day culture period, increased proportions of human PBMC expressed the alpha chain IL-2 receptor in response to IL-2 dose reduction from 1,000 (2 days) international units (IU) to 1 (4 days) IU per ml of cell culture (C), when compared against 6 days at 1,000 IU/ml (A), 6 days at 1 IU/ml (D), and 4 and 2 days at 1,000/ml and 1 IU/ml, respectively (B).

Multiple in vivo and in vitro models have been reported in support of a non-linear dose response curve when employing other cytokines (e.g., IFN-α, IFN-β, IFN-γ) alone or in combination with IL-2 (e.g., IL-2/IFN-α, IL-2/IFN-β, IL-2/IFN-γ, IL-2/TNF and IL-2/IL-4) (Table 1). In addition, based on experimental studies, both additive and synergistic modes of action have been hypothesized for IL-2 when combined with other biologic agents (Tables 2 through 6). Despite our lack of an in depth understanding of these cytokines and their physiological regulation [74, 82, 109, 123, 135, 147, 161] in vivo, recent advances in protein chemistry and recombinant technology have facilitated their broad clinical use as immunotherapeutic agents in advanced human malignancy.

Interleukin-2 based therapies in man have provided objective remissions associated with prolonged survival in advanced renal cell carcinoma and malignant melanoma [21, 45, 53, 136-139, 164, 165]. While these initial results have been promising, the clinical use of IL-2 alone and with other cytokines has raised the following questions regarding the role and potential benefit of

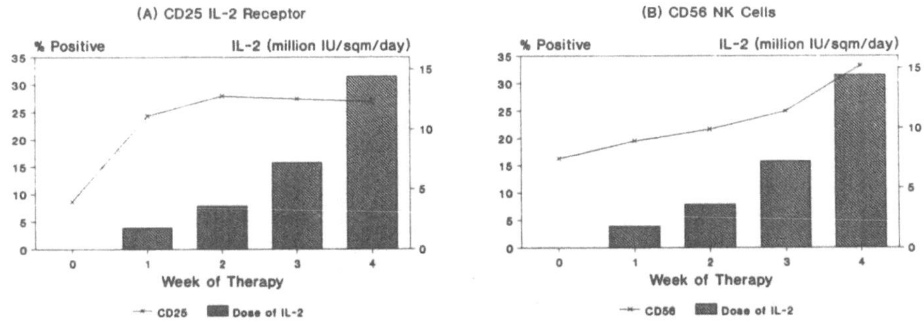

Figure 2. In vivo upregulation of Alpha Chain IL-2 receptor (CD25) positive lymphocytes and natural killer (NK/CD56) cells in response to the systemic administration of subcutaneous (SC) Recombinant IL-2.]
SC IL-2 was administered every twelve hours at escalating doses between 1.8 million international units (IU) per m² per day (week 1) and 14.4 million IU per m² per day (week 4); CD25 and CD56 cell surface expression of circulating patient lymphocytes was measured by FACS fluorescence analysis using specific monoclonal antibodies. Upon dose escalation of SC IL-2, a non-linear (A) and linear (B) dose response curve was observed for IL-2 receptor positive lymphocytes and NK cells, respectively.

biologic response modifiers in antineoplastic therapy:

1. How can we optimize the 'therapeutic index' of IL-2 based immunotherapy?
2. While dose escalation of IL-2 eventually produces severe and life-threatening toxicity, does it also improve its therapeutic efficacy?
3. How can we define the 'optimal' biological response modifying dose for IL-2 based immunotherapy in man?
4. Can we employ cytokine therapy in an effort to provide for a survival benefit of patients with advanced malignancy without compromising quality of life in the palliative situation?
5. What is the potential role for IL-2 based immunotherapy in combined modality approaches, e.g. for the treatment of residual disease after chemotherapy, and for disease prevention in the surgical adjuvant setting?

Rationales for combination therapy

Combination therapy may present the logical answer to limited efficacy of single agents. Its promise is essentially based on three hypotheses for the selection of a cytokine best combined with IL-2: (a) the potential combination agent by itself exhibits significant antitumour activity; (b) the additional agent stimulates the immune response via different and eventually synergistic biologic mechanisms thus evoking a more potent immune stimulation and antitumour activity with no evidence of cross resistance; (c) combination therapy improves the therapeutic index and cost benefit ratio in the tumour patients treated.

If IL-2 based treatment regimens are to operate via secondary cytokines in

Table 1. Selected in-vivo and in-vitro models supporting a non-linear dose response curve

		Ref
IL-2	– in vivo induction of T lymphocyte subsets upon IV bolus IL-2 in cancer patients with maximum increases at 4.0-8.9 MU/sqm and less potent stimulation at 10.0-14.0 MU/sqm	[62]
	– maximum in vivo immunostimulation in patients treated with IL-2 at doses below the maximum tolerated dose with a plateau in lymphocyte counts starting at 16.0 MU/sqm	[49]
	– inverse correlation between therapeutic antitumour activity in vivo and LAK activity in the presence of low IL-2 concentrations compared to increased IL-2 doses	[33]
	– higher anti-tumour efficacy of cells generated from tumour draining lymph nodes from mice cultured in 0.1-1.0 ng/ml of IL-2 compared to 10 ng/ml	[98]
IFN-α	– inverse correlation between cytokine dose and in vivo NK activation in cancer patients	[46, 47]
	– inverse relation between augmentation of murine ex vivo LAK activity and cytokine dose	[32]
	– inverse correlation between cytokine dose and murine splenocyte proliferation	[79]
IFN-β	– maximum NK cytotoxicity potentiation of murine spleen cell populations in vitro at 1.0 MU/culture and less potent stimulation at higher concentrations	[91]
IFN-τ	– in vivo activation of blood monocytes to lyse autologous tumour in cancer patients by systemically administered low cytokine doses with less activation at high doses	[83]
	– inverse correlation between cytokine dose and antitumour activity against SC melanoma in mice	[141]
IL-2/IFN-α	– inverse correlation between IFN dose and ex vivo NK activity in patients receiving IL-2 and IFN-α	[27]
IL-2/IFN-β	– inverse correlation between IFN-β dose and ex vivo measured LAK generation	[87]
IL-2/IFN-γ	– maximum in vivo induction of LAK activity at 1.0-3.0 MU/sqm of IL-2 with dose escalation failing to further increase LAK activity when given combined with IFN-γ	[133]
	– maximum in vivo synergism against murine pulmonary MCA sarcoma metastases at an intermediate dosage with less efficacy at lower or higher doses	[4]
	– Lack of significant differences for IL-2 concentrations from 6,250 U to 25,000 U per injection when combined with IFN-γ in the therapy of melanoma bearing mice	[141]
IL-2/TNF	– inverse correlation between IL-2 concentration and in vitro synergy of TNF in cytotoxicity enhancement in human lymphocytes	[121]
IL-2/IL-4	– greater expansion of tumour infiltrating lymphocytes from melanoma patients maintained with IL-2 and IL-4 in subsequent culture with low-dose IL-2 compared to higher dosages of IL-2 and IL-4	[76]

Abbreviations: IL-2, interleukin-2; IFN-α, interferon-alpha; IFN-β, interferon-beta; IFN-γ, interferon-gamma; TNF, tumour necrosis factor; IL-4, interleukin-4; IV, intravenous; SC, subcutaneous; MU, million units; NK, natural killer cell; LAK, lymphokine activated killer cell.

Table 2. Interleukin-2 and Interferon-α: selected preclinical models

		Ref
In Vitro		
1981	additive augmentation of NK cytolytic activity in murine spleen cell cultures	[59]
1985	synergistic induction of NK activity in cloned CTL lines of mice	[23]
1985	augmentation of CTL cytotoxicity in NK-depleted murine spleen cells	[148]
1986	more than additive augmentation of NK activity, dose dependent inhibition of proliferation and LAK activity of murine spleen cells and hPBL	[25]
1987	increase in susceptibility to LAK mediated lysis of human melanoma cell lines	[43]
1988	enhancement of cell-mediated cytotoxicity of human plasma cell leukemia effector cells against autologous tumour cells	[4]
1988	stimulation of murine splenocyte proliferation at low IFN-α doses, inhibition at higher doses	[79]
1988	synergistic NK activation; antagonism on proliferation, LAK activity, and IL-2 receptor expression of hPBL	[142]
1989	antagonism on LAK activity generation and proliferation in hPBMC cultures	[155]
1990	increased susceptibility of tumour cells to LAK lysis in vitro by preincubation with IFN-α	[15]
1991	synergy in NK activation of isolated lung interstitial rat lymphocytes	[92]
Animal		
1987	synergistic antitumour effect on visceral and nonvisceral reticulum cell sarcoma metastases in mice, increased NK like activity in vivo	[26]
1987	synergistic antitumour activity against SC transplanted colon carcinoma in mice	[158]
1988	synergistic antitumour effect on murine hepatic sarcoma metastases, survival benefit over either cytokine alone	[29]
1988	synergistic T cell mediated antitumour effect on various syngeneic murine tumours	[68]
1988	therapeutic synergy against pulmonary fibrosarcoma metastases in mice	[80]
1988	therapeutic synergy against murine pulmonary sarcoma metastases	[137]
1989	synergy in tumour regression, prolongation of survival, and cure rates in SC and hepatic sarcoma metastases in mice	[103]
1990	synergistic reduction in tumour burden and increase in survival with induction of specific CTL against hepatic metastases of colonic adenocarcinoma in mice	[13]
1990	augmentation of LAK activity in the lungs and spleen of mice depending on IFN-α dose	[32]
1990	increase after initial inhibition of lymphoid cell proliferation in various organs of mice	[126]
1991	survival benefit in the therapy of pulmonary sarcoma metastases in mice	[81]
1991	synergistic enhancement of LAK lysis of sarcoma target cells in various murine organs	[127]

Abbreviations: NK, natural killer cell; CTL, cytotoxic T lymphocyte; LAK, lymphokine-activated killer cell; hPBL, human peripheral blood lymphocyte; SC, subcutaneous.

vivo [5], the deliberate exogenous administration of defined doses of these biologic agents in conjunction with IL-2 may be highly reasonable. Therefore, multiple preclinical models have been developed both in the test tube and in animals in an attempt to select candidates for IL-2 combination therapy.

Table 3. Interleukin-2 and Interferon-γ: selected preclinical models

		Ref
In Vitro		
1981	potentiation of NK cytotoxicity of murine splenocytes against YAC-lymphoma cells	[94]
1985	synergistic induction of NK activity in cloned CTL from mice	[23]
1986	synergistic augmentation of cytotoxicity of long-term T cell cultures against EBV transformed autologous B cells	[30]
1986	enhancement of cytolytic potential of T3-negative NK cell derived cell lines	[160]
1988	antagonism on proliferation, LAK activity and IL-2 receptor expression in hPBL	[142]
1988	enhancement of K 562 target lysis and of c-myb mRNA levels in a cloned line of human NK cells	[86]
1991	Lack of synergism on LAK response in homogenous T acute lymphocytic leukemia cells	[75]
1991	synergistic enhancement of NK activity of lung interstitial rat lymphocytes against YAC-1 target cells	[92]
Animal		
1986	synergistic regression of SC transplanted murine adenocarcinoma, lack of antitumour synergism in athymic mice	[67]
1988	potentiation of antitumour activity against SC adenocarcinoma in low NK activity beige mice	[68]

Abbreviations: NK, natural killer cell; CTL, cytotoxic T lymphocytes; SC, subcutaneous.

Interferon-alpha and Interleukin-2

Recombinant human interferon-alpha (IFN-α) is known to possess antiviral properties [69], to modulate cytolytic T cell activity [23, 148] and NK cell-mediated cytotoxicity [24, 46, 59, 60], to enhance expression of MHC [56, 65, 162] and tumour associated antigens [18, 56, 110], to inhibit the generation of suppressor cells [84], and to exert potent antiproliferative activity against some tumours [24, 128]. By itself, IFN-α has demonstrated clinical efficacy in various malignancies including hairy cell leukemia [31, 130], chronic myelogenous leukemia [152], lymphomas [99, 129], malignant melanoma [38, 95], and renal cell carcinoma [89, 111, 128].

In pre-clinical human and murine models (Table 2), IFN-α and IL-2 exhibited a dose-dependent synergistic activation of NK cells [4, 26, 29, 59], while antagonistic effects on IL-2 receptor expression and lymphocyte proliferation were observed [142, 154]. In preclinical animal models, IFN-α showed considerable therapeutic synergy with IL-2 against a broad variety of murine tumours [13, 29, 32, 81, 103, 137, 158] as shown in Table 2. In human, IFN-α presents the cytokine most often combined with IL-2 (Tables 7 and 8).

Table 4. Interleukin-2 and Interferon-γ: selected preclinical models

		Ref
In Vitro		
1984	more than additive increase in human NK cytotoxicity	[149]
1985	synergy in proliferation and LAK activity in human PBMC	[70]
1985	augmentation of TNF-α and TNF-β production in human PBMC	[114]
1985	enhancement of TNF-β production by hPBMC, earlier appearance and augmented production of TNF mRNA	[150]
1986	enhancement of NK activity	[20]
1986	increase of LAK activity in murine splenocytes; more than additive increase in NK activity and enhancement of LAK activity in human PBL	[25]
1987	augmentation of IL-2 receptor expression in human PBMC	[40]
1988	lack of effects on LAK induction, lymphocyte proliferation, and IL-2 receptor expression in human lymphocyte cultures	[142]
1989	weak synergy in IL-2 and TNF-α production in monocytes	[61]
1989	augmentation or suppression of LAK induction, depending on the presence of adherent mononuclear cells	[156]
1990	synergistic induction of TNF-α mRNA in murine peritoneal macrophages	[142]
1990	stimulation of murine macrophage antimicrobial activity	[14]
1990	costimulation of the induction of murine macrophage tumouricidal activity	[36]
1991	less than additive enhancement of IL-1 production, synergistic enhancement of IL-1 secretion and TNF-α production by peripheral blood monocytes	[39]
1991	synergy with low levels of IL-2 to promote LAK differentiation in homogenous T leukemic preparations and in human PBL	[75]
Animal		
1988	synergistic effect in the therapy of NK resistant pulmonary sarcoma metastases	[1]
1988	lack of synergy against hepatic sarcoma metastases in mice	[29]
1988	synergistic reduction of pulmonary sarcoma	[44]
1988	retardation of SC adenocarcinoma growth in mice	[68]
1988	additive antitumour effects against SC tumours; synergistic antitumour effects against IP tumours in a murine melanoma system	[141]
1991	lack of additive effects in the therapy of intramammary implants of an immunogenic, syngeneic murine mammary carcinoma	[159]
1991	synergy in ex vivo LAK activity induction in murine organs	[127]

Abbreviations: NK, natural killer cell; LAK, lymphokine activated killer cell; PBMC, peripheral blood mononuclear cell; PBL, peripheral blood lymphocyte; SC, subcutaneous; IP, intraperitoneal.

Interferon-beta and Interleukin-2

Recombinant human interferon-beta (IFN-β) and IFN-α bind to the same cell surface receptor [2]. Both cytokines are thought to exert overlapping biologic effects [12]; thus, direct anti-proliferative and potent immunomodulatory activities [56] have been reported, including the augmentation of NK [24, 60] and cytotoxic T lymphocyte (CTL) functions [23]. In animal models, IFN-β has shown significant antitumour activity [94]; it synergizes with IL-2 in the

Table 5. Interleukin-2 and TNF-α: selected preclinical models

		Ref
In Vitro		
1987	augmentation of NK and LAK activity in nonadherent human PBL when combined with low dose IL-2; increased induction of IL-2 receptor expression on purified CD16 positive LGL	[119]
1988	synergy in LAK generation in human LGL preparations with low concentrations of IL-2, which were ineffective by themselves	[34]
1988	synergy with suboptimal levels of IL-2 in the generation of LAK activity in human PBMC	[48]
1988	augmentation of NK and LAK generation in human PBMC at levels equivalent to 10-fold higher concentrations of IL-2 when used alone	[121]
1989	induction of high-affinity IL-2 receptor expression exclusively in LGL upon stimulation with combined IL-2/TNF; augmentation of LAK induction in LGL precursors in the presence of suboptimal IL-2 concentrations	[17]
1989	augmentation of LAK induction; increased lymphocyte-mediated oncolytic activity against fresh primary lung carcinoma targets when compared to IL-2 alone	[169]
1990	enhancement of NK and LAK function in human PBMC from patients treated with IL-2/IFN-α	[51]
1991	synergy in IL-1 secretion, less than additive enhancement of IL-1 production by peripheral blood monocytes	[39]
1991	inhibition of PMN-phagocytosis by human PBMC	[107]
1991	synergistic NK activation in lung interstitial rat lymphocytes	[92]
Animal		
1987	synergistic antitumour effects resulting in the cure of a majority of lymphoma bearing mice; acquisition of systemic and permanent immunity against reinjected tumour cells	[116]
1987	antitumour synergy against SC experimental tumours in mice; synergy required TNF at MTD, whereas IL-2 dose could be reduced to 10% of MTD	[168]
1988	synergistic antitumour effects against immunogenic sarcoma in mice measured by tumour regression, cure rates, and prolongation of survival; maximum synergy upon triple combination of IL-2/TNF-α/IFN-α	[102]
1991	lack of additive effects on in vivo LAK induction in mice	[127]

Abbreviations: NK, natural killer cell; LAK, lymphokine activated killer cell; LGL, large granular lymphocyte; PBMC, peripheral blood mononuclear cell; PMN, polymorphonuclear cell; MTD, maximum tolerated dose.

induction of murine and human NK and CTL activity (Table 3).

As shown in Table 9, three phase I IL-2/IFN-β trials were reported in advanced human malignancies. Zamkoff [171] and Paolozzi [124] observed dose limiting toxicites including fever, hypotension, and skin reactions. No major response occurred; stabilization of disease was attained in 24% of a total of 50 advanced cancer patients with unreported diagnoses.

In a phase I study, Krigel et al. [87] observed fatigue, anorexia/weight loss, arthralgias, and depression as major side effects of combination therapy; a partial remission was reported in one out of three melanoma patients, and 3

Table 6. Interleukin-2 and Interleukin-4: selected preclinical models

		Ref
In Vitro		
1987	evidence for augmentation of LAK activity in murine splenocytes against syngeneic, NK resistant sarcoma targets	[108]
1987	dose-dependent antagonism on LAK generation against Daudi and melanoma target cells; additive or synergistic promotion of T cell growth	[144]
1987	antagonism on lytic effector cell activity in human PBL	[167]
1988	inhibition of LAK generation and function in human PBL against ovarian tumour cell lines	[54]
1988	inhibition of proliferation and differentiation of IL-2 stimulated B cells	[71]
1988	augmentation of tumour infiltrating T lymphocyte growth specific to autolgous melanoma; inhibition of nonspecific LAK activity from lymphocytes by inhibition of precursor cells	[76]
1988	dose-dependent antagonism on human LAK activity but not on NK activity	[55]
1988	antagonism on proliferation of monoclonal B cells	[73]
1988	inhibition of proliferation, but not differentiation of activated human B cells	[42]
1988	inhibition of human LAK activity, but not of the generation of antigen-specific CTL in mixed leukocyte cultures	[145]
1989	suppression of immunoglobulin production by IL-2 stimulated B cells depending on the activator used to stimulate B cells	[146]
1989	dose-dependent antagonism on proliferation and LAK activity from unstimulated PBMC; augmentation of proliferation and LAK activity from in vitro IL-2 preactivated PBMC	[77]
1989	augmentation of LAK induction in in vivo activated PBL from some IL-2 treated patients	[63]
1990	inhibition of proliferation in normal PBMC, augmentation of proliferation in PBMC from some IL-2 treated patients	[157]
1990	antagonism of LAK generation, DNA synthesis, IL-2 receptor expression, TNF-α and IFN-γ production by human PBL	[22]
1990	in vitro antagonism on NK and LAK activity by PBMC from patients treated with IL-2/IFN-α	[50]
1990	inhibition of TNF production in murine mononuclear phagocytes	[101]
1990	reduction of IL-2 receptor expression and antagonism on proliferation of human peripheral blood T cells stimulated with low dose anti-CD3	[100]
1991	augmentation of proliferative response of normal and leukemic CD3 positive LGL	[3]
1991	antagonism on NK cytolytic activity in LGL; synergistic suppression of immunoglobulin synthesis stimulated human PBL	[19]
1991	dose-dependent inhibition of costimulatory action on tumouricidal activity in IFN-γ treated macrophages; reduction of macrophage IL-2 receptor α-chain mRNA expression	[37]
1991	augmentation of tumouricidal activity against fibrosarcoma cell lines by human cytolytic T lymphocytes from tumour draining lymph nodes	[98]
Animal		
1991	decrease of in vivo tumouricidal activity against murine fibrosarcoma after in vitro generation of CTL effector cells from tumour draining lymph nodes	[98]
1991	lack of effect on in vivo LAK induction in mice	[127]

Abbreviations: LAK, lymphokine activated killer cell; NK, natural killer cell; PBL, peripheral blood lymphocyte; CTL, cytotoxic T lymphocyte; PBMC, peripheral blood mononuclear cells; LGL, large granular lymphocyte.

Table 7. Interleukin-2 plus Interferon-α: phase I/II combination studies*

Investigator	Year	Phase	Mode of applic	Dose	Responders / Total (95% CI)		Response duration (months)+	Ref
					Renal carcinoma	Malignant melanoma		
rIL-2 IV Bolus								
Rosenberg et al	1989	I	IFN-α IL-2	IV 6 0)3 0-6 0) MU/sqm/8h IV 4 5 (1 0-4 5) MRU/SQM/8h	5/13 (14-68%)	6/14 (18-71%)	3-14+ #	[139]
Budd et al	1990	I	IFN-α IL-2	IM 0-10 0 MU/sqm/d x3/w IV 0 1-2 0 MBRMPU/sqm/d x3/w	1/12 (0-38%)	1/6 (0-64%)	1 5-3	[27]
Kruit et al	1991	II	IFN-α IL 2	IV 3 0 MU/sqm/d x5/w IV 4 5 MBRMPU/sqm/8h	0/0	5/9 (21 86%)	-	[90]
rIL-2 Constant IV Infusion								
Lee et al	1989	I	IFN-α IL-2	IM 5 0 (2 0-10 0) MU/sqm/d IV 3 0 (1 0-3 0) MRU/sqm/d	0/2 (0-84%)	3/7 (10-82%)	3+ #	[93]
Bergmann et al	1990	I/II	IFN-α IL-2	SQ 10 0 MU/sqm/d x7/w CI 18 0 MIU/sqm/d$	2/5 (5-85%)	3/11 (6-61%)	-	[16]
Bukowski et al	1990	I	IFN-α IL-2	IM 5 0-10 0 MU/sqm/d x3/w CI 3 0-4 5 MBRMPU/sqm/d x5/w	3/7 (10-82%)	0/0	-	[28]
Hirsch et al	1990	I	IFN α IL 2	IM 3 0-12 0 MU/sqm/d x3/w CI 1 0-2 0 MRU/sqm/d x5/w	6/12 (21-79%)	0/3 (0 71%)	12+-19+	[64]
Huberman et al	1991	I	IFN-α IL 2	IM 6 0 MU/sqm/d x3/w 2hIV 4 0 (1 0-4 0) MRU/sqm/d x5/w	0/2 (0-84%)	1/5 (1-72%)	3+	[66]
Keilholz et al	1991	II	IFN α IL-2	SQ 10 0 MU/sqm/d x5/w CI 0 25 mg/sqm/d-1 0 mg/sqm/6h	0/0	9/22 (21-64%)	-	[78]
Kruit et al	1991	II	IFN-α IL-2	SQ 6 0 MU/sqm/d x2/w CI 3 0 MBRMPU/sqm/d x4/w	0/0	11/54 (11-34%)	4 8+ &	[90]
Pichert et al	1991	II	IFN-α IL 2	SQ 6 0 MU/sqm/d x2/w CI 3 0 MRU/sqm/d x4/w	0/6 (0-46%)	2/8 (1-35%)	1-7	[125]
Figlin et al	1992	II	IFN α IL 2	IM/SQ 6 0 MU/sqm/d x2/w CI 2 0 MRU/sqm/d x4/w	9/30 (15-49%)	0/0	12+ &	[52]
rIL-2 SQ Injection								
Atzpodien et al	1990	I	IFN-α IL-2	SQ 5 0 MU/sqm x3/w SQ 1 8-9 0 MIU/sqm/12h x5/w	5/14 (13 65%)	1/7 (0-58%)	4+ 8 5+	[6]
Atzpodien et al	1991	I/II	IFN-α IL-2	SQ 3 0-6 0 MU/sqm x3/w SQ 3 6-4 8 MIU/sqm/d x5/w	14/50 (16-42%)	0/0	23+ #	[8]
Sznol et al	1991	I	IFN-α IL 2	SQ 1 5-3 0 MU/sqm/d x3/w SQ 1 5-3 0 MRU/sqm/d x5/w	5/–	0/12 (0 26%	-	[154]

* The majority of investigators conducted dose-escalation trials, in some studies, the 'optimal' therapeutic dose level is quoted, dose ranges given in parentheses

\+ Median or range given

\# Duration of complete responses

& Duration of partial responses

$ In renal cancer patients, an escalated 1-hour-infusion regimen was applied

Abbreviations Applic, application, CI, confidence interval, IFN-α, recombinant human interferon-alpha2, IL 2, recombinant human interleukin 2, IV, intravenous bolus infusion, IM, intramuscular, SQ, subcutaneous, CI, constant intravenous infusion, MU, million units, MRU, million Roche units, MIU, million international units, MBRMPU, million Biological Response Modifiers Program units

minor remissions occurred; one out of one remission was seen in a patient with carcinoid tumour, one out of one in metastatic synovial sarcoma, and one out of three in metastatic melanoma; 66% of all evaluable patients presented with stable disease after 4 weeks of therapy.

Table 8. Interleukin-2 plus Interferon-α: toxicity upon systemic therapy

Toxicity	Grade III / IV (%)*		
	IL-2 Dose Level / Mode of Application		
	Low dose SC+	Intermediate dose/IV #	high dose/IV&
Fever/Malaise	5	60	100
Fluid Retention/Weight Gain	0	33	n.r.
Nausea/Vomiting	2	n.r.	100
Hypotension	0	60	n.r.
Dyspnoea/Respiratory Distress	2	27	n.r.
Hepatic Toxicity	2	3	15
Renal Toxicity	0	20	22
Neurologic Toxicity	0	13	36
Anemia	0	20	n.r.
Thrombocytopenia	0	22	n.r.
Granulocytopenia	0	n.r.	50

* Toxicity grading was adapted from the WHO scale. Maximum percentages are given.
\+ Studies reported: Atzpodien [8].
\# Studies reported: Hirsch [64], Huberman [66], Mittelman [105], Kruit [90], Lee [98], Pichert [128].
& Studies reported: Kruit [90], Rosenberg [139].
Abbreviations: IL-2, recombinant human interleukin-2; n.r., not reported.

Tamura et al. [153] described dose-limiting fatigue and hepatotoxicity; one minor remission among two patients with metastatic pharyngeal cancer was reported.

In a published phase II trial [88], response rates in renal cell carcinoma were well in the range of responses observed upon IL-2/IFN-α combination therapy (Table 7); IL-2 and IFN-β were administered as 1 minute IV bolus each, three times weekly for 4 weeks. Therapy was well tolerated in the outpatient setting. In 22 evaluable renal cancer patients, one complete, five partial, and three minor remissions were reported, rendering this treatment modality a markedly promising one [88].

Interferon-gamma and Interleukin-2

Recombinant human interferon-gamma (IFN-γ) as single agent is known to enhance NK [132], T cell [30], and monocyte cytotoxicity [113, 122], and to induce IL-2 receptor expression on NK cells [70]; it may also modulate expression of other cell surface molecules including tumour associated antigens [110], and MHC antigens [65, 85, 120].

As shown in Table 4, upon combination with IL-2, IFN-γ synergistically enhanced IL-2 induced lymphocyte proliferation, NK and LAK activity, TNF-α and IL-1 secretion, and expression of IL-2 receptors on human peripheral blood

Table 9. Interleukin-2 plus other Cytokines: Phase I/II Combination Studies

Cytokine	Investigator	Year	Phase	n	Mode of Applic.	Dose	Ref
IFN-β	Krigel et al	1988	I	47	IFN-β IV	2.0-20.0 MU/sqm	[87]
					IL-2 SQ/IV	0,06-30.0 MIU/sqm	
	Paolozzi et al.	1989	I	50	IFN-β IV	2.0-10.0 MU/sqm	[124]
					IL-2 SQ	0.06-30.0 MIU/sqm	
	Tamura et al.	1989	I	26	IFN-β IV	0.1-6.0 MU/sqm	[153]
					IL-2 CI	0.33 - 1.7 MIU	
	Krigel et al.	1990	II	22	IFN-β IV	6.0 MU/sqm	[88]
					IL-2 IV	30.0 MIU/sqm	
IFN-γ	Farace et al.	1990	I	29	IFN-γ IV	2.0 MU/sqm*	[49]
					IL-2 CI	1.0-24.0 MIU/sqm	
	Redman et al.	1990	I	26	IFN-γ IM	25.0-750.0 μg/sqm	[133]
					IL-2 CI	6.0 - 18.0 MIU/sqm	
	Weiner et al.	1991	I	41	IFN-γ SQ	10.0-250.0 μg/sqm	[163]
					IL-2 IV	6.0 - 45.0 MIU/sqm	
	Baars et al.	1991	I	32	IFN-γ IM	10.0-100.0 μg/sqm	[11]
					IL-2 IV	3.0 - 18.0 MIU/sqm	
TNF-α	Rosenberg et al.	1989	I/II	38	TNF-α IV	50.0-350.0 μg/sqm	[138]
					IL-2 IV	0.18 - 0.6 MIU/kg	
	West et al.	1989	I	-	TNF-α CI	60.0 μg/sqm	[166]
					IL-2 CI	18.0 MIU/sqm	
	Yang et al.	1991	I	16	TNF-α IM	25.0-100.0 μg/sqm	[170]
					IL-2 CI	6.0 MIU/sqm	
IL-4	Netaji et al.	1991	I	11	IL-4 SQ	40.0-400.0 μg/sqm	[115]
					IL-2 IV	1.0 - 16.0 MU/sqm	
	Olencki et al.	1991	I	27	IL-4 SQ	40.0-400.0 μg/sqm	[118]
					IL-2 IV	1.0 - 16.0 MU/sqm	

* Patients received IFn-γ over 5 consecutive days, before receiving IL-2.
Abbreviations: n, number of patients; Applic., applications; IFN-β, recombinant human interferon-beta; IL-2, recombinant human interleukin-2; IFN-γ, recombinant human interferon-gamma; TNF-α, recombinant human tumour necrosis factor-alpha; IL-4, recombinant human interleukin-4; IV, intravenous bolus infusion; SQ, subcutaneous; CI, constant intravenous infusion; IM, intramuscular; MU, million units; MIU, million international units.

mononuclear cells. In the murine model, the combination of IL-2/IFN-γ demonstrated schedule dependent induction of ex vivo NK activity, differential effects on LAK activity, and occasional synergism in some experimental tumours (Table 4).

Four phase I trials employing IL-2/IFN-γ combination therapy were reported in human (Table 9). According to the regimen by Farace et al. [49], IV IL-2 was preceded by a 5-day course of IFN-γ infusions; IFN-γ had no significant effect on IL-2 induced immune stimulation. Four partial remissions were obtained in a total of 15 patients with metastastic melanoma, and one partial regression occurred among 6 renal cancer patients.

Redman et al. [133] reported dose limiting toxicities including respiratory distress upon IL-2/IFN-γ combination therapy. Objective clinical responses in 26 evaluable patients included a partial remission in one of four patients with non-Hodgkin's lymphoma, a minor remission in one of six patients with renal cell carcinoma, and mixed responses in another three patients.

Weiner et al. [163] observed fatigue and non-specific side effects; however, in the absence of grade 3 or 4 toxicities, the maximum tolerated dose was not attained in this trial. After six weeks of therapy, among 33 patients evaluable for response, one of 12 renal carcinoma patients and one of 7 metastatic melanoma patients presented with partial remission; and minor responses were seen in two patients.

Baars et al. [11] reported dose-limiting hypotension and hepatotoxicity upon IL-2/IFN-γ combination therapy. Among 23 evaluable patients, one patient each with metastatic renal cancer and with metastatic melanoma achieved a partial remission (Table 9).

tumour necrosis factor-alpha and Interleukin-2

Recombinant human tumour necrosis factor-alpha (TNF-α) is known to induce the growth of various human cell lines including cloned human fibroblasts. It has also been shown to support development of cytotoxic T lymphocytes [131], and to enhance cytotoxic activity of NK cells [119]. In vivo, TNF-α caused haemorrhagic necrosis of tumour grafts in mice [58].

Upon combination with IL-2, TNF-α was shown to synergistically enhance NK and LAK activity and to modulate secretion of IL-1 by human peripheral blood cells in vitro (Table 5). In the murine model, IL-2/TNF-α combination therapy resulted in synergistic antitumour effects; in addition, extension of survival and complete tumour regressions were observed (Table 5).

Three clinical trials employing IL-2/TNF-α combination therapy were reported (Table 9). Rosenberg et al. [138] observed dose limiting WHO grade IV hypotension upon combined high dose IV IL-2/TNF-α treatment; among a total of 37 evaluable patients, one of 15 patients with metastatic melanoma achieved a CR, and 3 PR occurred in a total of 10 patients with metastatic renal cell cancer.

West et al. employed sequential administration of IL-2 and TNF-α via continuous infusion [166]. While therapeutic efficacy in malignant melanoma and renal cell cancer was comparable to single agent IL-2, one PR each occurred in a patient with adenocarcinoma of the lung, and in a colorectal carcinoma patient.

In a series of 16 patients with non-small cell lung cancer who received low-dose IL-2/TNF-α combination therapy [170], one PR and 3 MR were noted among 12 evaluable patients.

Interleukin-4 and Interleukin-2

Recombinant human interleukin-4 (IL-4) was previously found to modulate the growth of stimulated B cells [35, 73, 117]. It also augments MHC class II antigen expression, enhances immunoglobulin production, stimulates the growth of some T cells and mast cell lines; in addition, it has been shown to support the development of cytotoxic T lymphocytes [54, 55, 76, 73, 98, 104, 106, 146, 167]. Interleukin-2 and IL-4 synergize in the activation and proliferation of MHC restricted CTL, whereas IL-4 may antagonize IL-2 mediated LAK generation (Table 6). There are only a limited number of reports studying the IL-2/IL-4 combination in animal models as summarized in Table 6.

In preliminary reports from IL-2/IL-4 combination trials in humans, no major antitumour effects have been reported yet (Table 9). Major toxicities upon combination therapy included serum alkaline phosphatase elevations and cardiac arrhythmias as reported by Netaji et al. [115], furthermore marked monocytosis, basophilia, and eosinophilia as reported by Olencki et al. [118]. Dose escalation studies are presently ongoing.

Interleukin-2 and interferon-α combination trials in advanced malignancy

IFN-α is the cytokine most widely used in combination trials with IL-2. Table 7 summarizes 16 clinical trials wherein a total of 528 advanced tumour patients received IL-2 and IFN-α. Considering 147 metastatic renal cell cancer and 72 metastatic malignant melanoma patients at the most effective dose levels, overall response rates of 26.5% (renal cell cancer; 95% confidence intervals, 0%-84%) and 18.1% (malignant melanoma; 95% confidence intervals, 0%-82%) were calculated. Reported response duration ranged from 1 month [125] to 23+ months [8]. While patient cohorts in these clinical phase I or II studies were usually small, it appeared that IL-2/IFN-α combination therapy in metastatic renal cell cancer was more effective than the most aggressive single agent regimen employing IL-2 (18% partial/complete remissions) [138] or IFN-α (17% partial/complete remissions) [111], respectively.

Over an IL-2 dose range from 3.6 million international units per m^2 per day [6] to 13.5 million Roche units per m^2 per day [139], no linear increase in therapeutic efficacy against metastatic renal cell carcinoma occurred when combining IL-2 with IFN-α at a standard dose of 5 to 6 million U per m^2 given thrice weekly up to every 8 hours. Thus, dose response correlation demonstrated 'optimal' therapeutic response to IL-2 at systemic doses up to 20-fold below the maximum tolerated dose defined previously [136].

The mode of application of IL-2 had no significant impact on therapeutic efficacy, whereby thrice daily intravenous bolus as pioneered by Rosenberg and colleagues [136], 24 hour constant intravenous infusion developed by West et al. [165] and subcutaneous administration of IL-2 [6] yielded comparable results in patients with metastatic renal cell carcinoma.

In a prospective clinical trial conducted at our institution, combination immunotherapy employing subcutaneous IL-2 and IFN-α could significantly extend survival in patients with advanced renal cell carcinoma when compared against untreated historic controls; thus, in a cohort of 50 outpatients, median survival from start of therapy was calculated at 20+ months [8]. Size of metastatic lesions was an independent prognostic parameter whereby patients with a maximum tumour diameter of 2 cm or less had a significantly longer survival from start of therapy than patients with lesions of more than 2 cm in diameter ($p<0.005$; Figure 3).

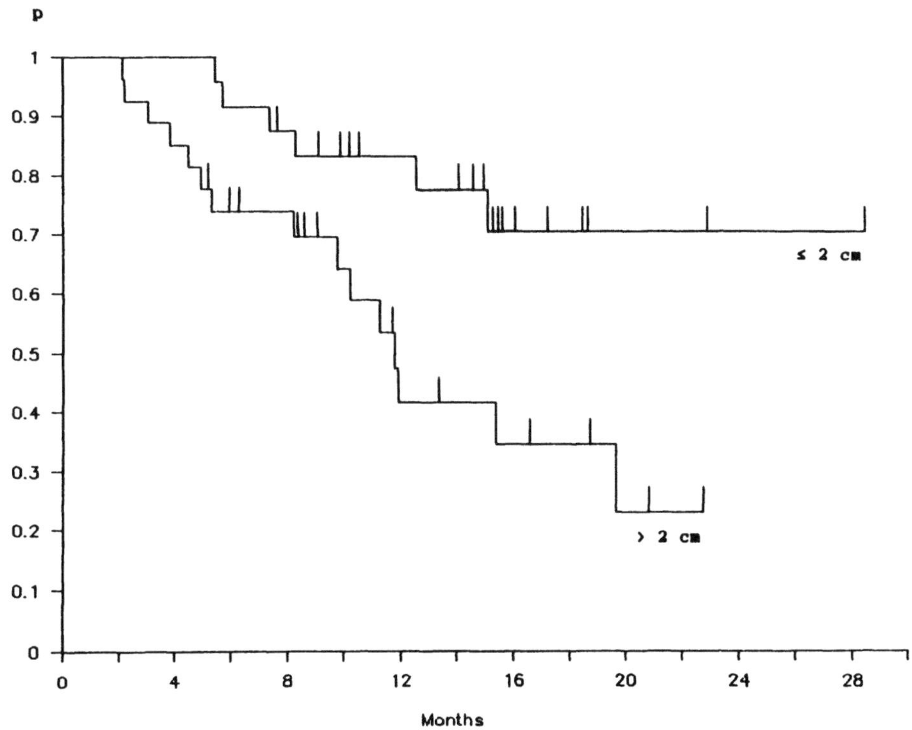

Figure 3. Survival Probability (Kaplan-Meier) from Start of Therapy in Metastatic Progressive Renal Cell Carcinoma Patients Receiving Subcutaneous (SC) Recombinant IL-2 and IFN-α. Survival Probability was compared in two separate cohorts of patients, who presented with maximum lesion size of ≤ 2 cm and > 2 cm, respectively; significance levels were calculated at $p < 0.05$.

While few tumour patients responding to recombinant cytokine therapy have had extensive disseminated disease, it is hypothesized that immunotherapy using IL-2 and/or IFN-α may be most effective in patients presenting with low tumour burden.

Quality of life and systemic toxicity in palliative IL-2 combination therapy

At our institution, to assess quality of life in patients receiving subcutaneous IL-2 and IFN-α as home therapy [6, 8], the Winnipeg Functional Living Index for Cancer (FLIC) was employed before, during and after therapy. This index comprised twenty-two items related to physical well-being, impact of illness, treatment-related side effects, emotional state including depression and anxiety, patient sociability, family interaction, and expectation of therapy outcome; the FLIC was previously shown to have adequate content, construct, and concurrent validity as well as reliability [140].

When comparing FLIC pre and post treatment values, quality of life was not significantly affected by low dose outpatient IL-2/IFN-α combination therapy (Table 10); however, treatment response had an impact on quality of life assessment in that patients presenting with an objective response to therapy or with disease stabilization experienced a marked increase in overall well-being when compared to pre therapy status. In contrast, advanced tumour patients with continuous progressive disease exhibited a concomitant deterioration of quality of life throughout cytokine therapy (Table 10).

Upon IL-2/IFN-α combination therapy, the systemic toxicity spectrum included constitutional symptoms such as fever, profound fatigue, nausea and weight loss, some of which eventually required dose reductions and/or rest periods (Table 8). The toxicity profile of low dose therapy employing subcutaneous IL-2 and IFN-α in the home therapy setting [6, 8] was in marked contrast to toxicity patterns observed in various clinical trials using IFN-α in conjunction with intermediate or high dose intravenous IL-2 [64, 66, 90, 93, 105, 125, 139] (Table 8).

Upon IV IL-2, between 60% and 100% of patients treated developed grade III or IV fever and malaise (SC IL-2, 5%); one third of patients or more exhibited grade III or IV sequelae of IL-2 induced capillary leak (i.e., interstitial edema and/or hypotension) when receiving intravenous therapy as opposed to 0% in the subcutaneous treatment group (Table 8). While life-threatening adverse events such as acute respiratory distress or severe hypotension occurred in up to 10% of high or intermediate dose IV IL-2 patients, similar systemic toxicity was never observed with SC low dose IL-2. In addition, in the vast majority of IL-2/IFN-α patients, grade III or IV renal, hepatic and haematologic toxicity was associated with intravenous but not with subcutaneous therapy (Table 8).

Current and future prospects in IL-2 combination therapy

Based on the current clinical experience from IL-2 combination trials, cytokines including IL-2 and IFN-α are also used in conjunction with chemotherapy. Pioneering chemo-immunotherapy regimens have yielded challenging clinical results mostly in patients with metastatic malignant melanoma (Table 11); thus,

Table 10. Subcutaneous IL-2 plus IFN-α: quality of life assessment

	Functional Living Index Score	
Clinical Result	Day 0	Week 7
CR + PR	116	120
SD	94	100
PD	72	60
Total	93	95

To assess quality of life, the Functional Living Index - Cancer (Winnipeg) was employed. Mean scores before (day 0) and after (week 7) the first treatment cycle were calculated on a relative scale from 20 to 140.

both increased objective response rates of 35% up to 83% and extended response durations of more than 23 months have been reported (Table 11) [9, 57, 96, 134] as opposed to a median response duration of 4 to 6 months in malignant melanoma patients receiving chemotherapy, only.

Among the proposed mechanisms of synergy of interleukin-2 and chemotherapy in malignant melanoma is an alteration in pharmacokinetics of dacarbazine due to IL-2 mediated enhancement of capillary permeability. In addition, the sequential use of chemotherapy and IL-2/IFN-α in clinical trials has indicated that IL-2 based immunotherapy is active after the previous use of cytotoxic and potentially immunosuppressing agents; thus, it did not appear that chemotherapy as used in these trials may abrogate response to subsequent IL-2. Moreover, in the majority of malignant melanoma patients reported, there was no clinical evidence of cross resistance between cytotoxic and biologic therapy.

In patients with progressive metastatic colorectal cancer, we conducted a phase I/II trial employing a combination of IL-2, IFN-α and 5-fluorouracil [10]. Response to this combination therapy (29% partial responders) was not significantly different from results obtained with 5-fluorouracil as single agent (Table 11).

While the combination of IL-2 based immunotherapy and chemotherapy may allow for a further improvement of the therapeutic index and cost benefit ratio in advanced tumour patients, the optimal design of combination regimens is subject to a plethora of further clinical and preclinical investigations. While immunotherapy employing the IL-2/IFN-α combination has replaced conventional cytotoxic agents in some tumours, it may also supplement conventional chemotherapy in the post remission induction and minimal residual disease settings. Therefore, augmentation of chemotherapy by IL-2 has become a major focus of current research.

Table 11. Interleukin-2 / Interferon-α: chemotherapy phase I/II combination studies

Investigator	Year	Combination	Responders / Total (95% CI) Malignant melanoma	Responders / Total (95% CI) Colorectal carcinoma	Response duration (months)*	Ref
Hamblin et al.	1991	DTIC + DDP	10/12 (52-98%)		14+ #	[57]
Legha et al.	1991	DTIC + DDP + VBL	13/35 (21-55%)		7+ &	[96]
Richards et al.	1991	DTIC + DDP + BCNU + TAM	20/34 (41-75%) $		-	[134]
Atzpodien et al.	1992	DTIC + CBDCA	14/40 (21-52%)		3-23+	[9]
Atzpodien et al.	1992	5-FU		4/14 (8-58%)	5.9	[10]

* Median or range given.
# Duration in the only complete responder not presenting with early CNS relapse.
& Median response duration in 8 of 13 responders.
$ Of 42 patients, 34 were evaluable for response after 1 cycle of treatment.
Abbreviations: CI, confidence interval; DTIC, dacarbazine; DDP, cisplatin; VBL, vinblastine; BCNU, carmustine; TAM, tamoxifen; CBDCA, carboplatin; 5-FU, 5-fluorouracil.

Summary

The use of recombinant human interleukin-2 alone or with other cytokines has given evidence of a non-linear dose response curve. This allows for optimal biological and therapeutic effects of IL-2 at dosages far below the maximum tolerated dose [6, 33, 49, 62, 74, 97, 98]. In recent IL-2 combination trials, both improved therapeutic response and extended progression free survival and/or overall survival have been reported when reducing IL-2 doses by more than 90% of the maximum tolerated dose and combining IL-2 with other agents (Table 7).

Significant enhancement of the therapeutic index of IL-2 in advanced cancer patients has been achieved through additive and potentially synergistic effects of IL-2 when used in conjunction with other cytokines, primarily with IFN-α. For the future design of IL-2 based clinical combination trials, however, the following issues remain open: (a) Which models favour concomitant versus sequential use of combination agents? (b) Which dose intensity and dose distribution will allow for the best therapeutic effect given a non-linear versus linear dose response curve? (c) Can IL-2 combination therapy be used in an effort to effectively overcome tumour resistance toward single agents/ (d) Why do different sites of metastatic disease respond differently to IL-2 therapy? (e) In which state of disease will patients benefit most from IL-2 combination therapy?

In addition, future clinical trials employing IL-2 in combination with other agents ought to resolve the following issues: (a) randomized trials are needed to provide conclusive evidence for an IL-2 related advantage in progression free and overall survival; (b) the clinical use of IL-2 combination therapy in tumour free patients status post surgery and/or in patients with minimal residual disease needs to be evaluated with regard to the potential role of IL-2 in the early disease setting.

References

1. Agah R, Malloy B, Sherrod A, Mazumder A. Successful therapy of natural killer-resistant pulmonary metastases by the synergism of γ-interferon with tumour necrosis factor and interleukin-2 in mice. Cancer Res 1988; 48: 2245-8.
2. Aguet M, Mogensen KE. Interferon receptors. In: Gresser I, (editor). Interferon 3. New York: Academic Press, 1983: 1-22.
3. Aprile JA, Russo M, Pepe MS, Loughran TP. Activation signals leading to proliferation of normal and leukemic CD3+ large granular lymphocytes. Blood 1991; 78: 1282-5.
4. Atzpodien J, Shimazaki C, Wisniewski D, et al. Interleukin-2 und Interferon-α in der adoptiven Immuntherapie des Plasmozytoms: Ein experimentelles Modell. In: Lutz D, Heinz R, Nowotny H, Stacher A, et al. (editors). Leukämien und Lymphome. München, Wien, Baltimore: Urban & Schwarzenberg 1988: 211-2.
5. Atzpodien J, Kirchner H. Cancer, cytokines, and cytotoxic cells: Interleukin-2 in the immunotherapy of human neoplasms. Klin Wochenschr 1990; 68: 1-11.
6. Atzpodien J, Körfer A, Franks CR, et al. Home therapy with recombinant interleukin-2 and interferon-α2b in advanced human malignancies. Lancet 1990; 335: 1509-12.
7. Atzpodien J, Poliwoda H, Kirchner H. Alpha-interferon and interleukin-2 in renal cell carcinoma: Studies in nonhospitalized patients. Semin Oncol 1991; 18: 108-12.
8. Atzpodien J, Körfer A, Schomburg A, et al. Outpatient treatment of metastatic renal cell carcinoma patients: Interleukin-2 in combination with interferon-α. Ann Oncol, 1992. In press.
9. Atzpodien J, Kirchner H, Schomburg A, et al. Outpatient chemo-immunotherapy of advanced malignant melanoma: sequential administration of sc interleukin-2 and interferon-α after iv dacarbazine and carboplatin. J Clin Oncol, 1992. In press.
10. Atzpodien J, Kirchner H, Körfer A, et al. Treatment of metastatic colorectal cancer patients with 5-fluorouracil in combination with recombinant subcutaneous human interleukin-2 and interferon-α. Oncol, 1992. In press.
11. Baars JW, Wagstaff J, Boven E, et al. Phase I study on the sequential administration of recombinant human Interferon-γ and recombinant human Interleukin-2 in patients with metastatic solid tumours. J Nat Cancer Inst, 1991; 83: 1408-10.
12. Balkwill FR. Peptid regulatory factors: Interferons. Lancet 1, 1989; 1060-3.
13. Bash JA, Arroyo PA, Wiegand G, et al. Direct effects of alpha interferon (IFN-α) on murine adenocarcinom C-C36 as a basis for synergy with interleukin-2 (IL-2) in cytolytic lymphocyte (CTL) mediated abrogation of hepatic metastases. Proc AACR 1990; 31: 251.
14. Belosevic M, Finbloom DS, Meltzer MS, Nacy CA. IL-2. A cofactor for induction of activated macrophage resistance to infection. J Immunol 1990; 145: 831-6.
15. Bergmann L, Weidmann E, Bungert B, et al. Influence of various cytokines on the induction of lymphokine-activated killer cells. Nat Immun Cell Growth Regul 1990; 9: 265-73.
16. Bergmann L, Weidmann E, Mitrou PS, et al. Interleukin-2 in combination with Interferon-alpha in disseminated malignant melanoma and advanced renal cell carcinoma. A phase I/II study. Onkologie 1990; 13: 137-40.
17. Blay JY, Bertoglio J, Fradelizi D, Chouaib S. Functional interactions of IL2 and TNF in the differentiation of LGL into LAK effectors. Int J Cancer 1989; 44: 598-604.
18. Borden EC. Augmented tumour-associated antigen expression by interferon. J Nat Cancer Inst 1988; 80: 8-14.

19. Bosse D, Ades E. Suppression of human immunoglobulin synthesis by Interleukin-4 in tandem with Interleukin-2 through large granular lymphocytes. Pathobiology 1991; 59: 391-5.
20. Braakman E, Van Tunen A, Meager A, Lucas CJ. IL-2- and IFNγ-enhanced natural cytotoxic activity: Analysis of the role of different lymphoid subsets and implications for activation routes. Cell Immunol 1986; 99: 476-88.
21. Bradley EC, Louie AC, Paradise CM, et al. Antitumour response in patients with metastatic renal cell carcinoma is dependent upon regimen intensity. Proc ASCO 1989; 8: 133.
22. Brooks B, Chapman K, Lawry J, et al. Suppression of lymphokine-activated killer (LAK) cell induction mediated by Interleukin-4 and transforming growth factor-β1: Effect of addition of exogenous tumour necrosis factor-alpha and Interferon-gamma, and measurement of their endogenous production. Clin Exp Immunol 1990; 82: 583-9.
23. Brooks CG, Holscher M, Urdal D. Natural killer activity in cloned cytotoxic T lymphocytes: Regulation by Interleukin 2, Interferon, and specific antigen. J Immunol 1985; 135: 1145-52.
24. Brunda MJ, Rosenbaum D, Stern L. Inhibition of experimentally-induced murine metastases by recombinant alpha interferon: correlation between the modulatory effect of interferon treatment on natural killer cell activity and inhibition of metastases. Int J Cancer 1984; 24: 421-6.
25. Brunda MJ, Tarnowski D, Davatelis V. Interaction of recombinant Interferons with recombinant Interleukin-2: Differential effects on natural killer cell activity and Interleukin-2-activated killer cells. Int J Cancer 1986; 37: 787-93.
26. Brunda MJ, Bellantoni D, Sulich V. In vivo anti-tumour activity of combinations of Interferon alpha and Interleukin-2 in a murine model. Correlation of efficacy with the induction of cytotoxic cells resembling natural killer cells. Int J Cancer 1987; 40: 365-71.
27. Budd GT, Osgood B, Barna B, et al. Phase I clinical trial of Interleukin 2 and α-Interferon: Toxicity and immunologic effects. Cancer Res 1989; 49: 6432-6.
28. Bukowski RM, Murthy S, Sergi J, et al. Phase I trial of continuous infusion recombinant Interleukin-2 and intermittent recombinant Interferon-alpha 2a: Clinical effects. J Biol Response Mod 1990; 9: 538-45.
29. Cameron RB, McIntosh JK, Rosenberg SA. Synergistic antitumour effects of combination immunotherapy with recombinant Interleukin-2 and a recombinant hybrid α-Interferon in the treatment of established murine hepatic metastases. Cancer Res 1988; 48: 5810-7.
30. Chen BP, Sondel PM. Cytotoxicity of autologous Epstein-Barr virus-transformed cells mediated by interleukin-2 dependent, long-term T cell cultures is augmented by beta, but not alpha, recombinant interferon. J Biol Response Mod 1986; 5: 351-61.
31. Cheson BD, Martin A. Clinical trials in hairy cell leukemia: current status and future directions. Ann Intern Med 1987; 106: 871-8.
32. Chikkala NF, Lewis I, Ulchaker J, et al. Interactive effects of α-Interferon A/D and Interleukin 2 on murine lymphokine-activated killer activity: Analysis at the effector and precursor level. Cancer Res 1990; 50: 1176-82.
33. Chou T, Chang AE, Shu S. Generation of therapeutic T lymphocytes from tumour-bearing mice by in vitro sensitization. J Immunol 1988; 140: 2453-61.
34. Chouaib S, Bertoglio J, Blay JY, et al. Generation of lymphokine-activated killer cells: Synergy between tumour necrosis factor and Interleukin 2. Immunology 1988; 85: 6875-9.
35. Coffman RL, Ohara J, Bond MW, et al. B cell stimulatory factor-1 enhances the IgE response of lipopolysaccharide-activated B cells. J Immunol 1986; 136: 4538-41.
36. Cox GW, Mathieson BJ, Giardina SL, Varesio L. Characterization of IL-2 receptor expression and function on murine macrophages. J Immunol 1990; 145: 1719-25.
37. Cox GW, Chattopadhyay U, Oppenheim JJ, Varesio L. IL-4 inhibits the costimulatory activity of IL-2 or picolinic acid but not of lipopolysaccharide on IFN-γ-treated macrophages. J Immunol 1991; 147: 3809-14.
38. Creagan ET, Ahmann DL, Green SJ. Phase II study of recombinant leukocyte alpha interferon in disseminated malignant melanoma. Cancer 1984; 54: 2844-9.
39. Danis VA, Franic GM, Rathjen DA, Brooks PM. Effects of granulocyte-macrophage colony-

stimulating factor (GM-CSF), IL-2, interferon-gamma (IFN-γ), tumour necrosis factor-alpha (TNF-α) and IL-6 on the production of immunoreactive Il-2 and TNF-α by human monocytes. Clin Exp Immunol 1991; 85: 143-450.
40. Daugherty JP, Weiner LM. Augmentation of IL-2-induced Il-2 receptor expression by IFN-δ. Proc AACR 1987; 28: 341.
41. DeFrance T, Vanbervliet B, Aubry J, et al. B cell growth-promoting activity of recombinant human interleukin-4. J Immunol 1987; 139: 1135-41.
42. DeFrance T, Vanbervliet B, Aubry J, Banchereau J. Interleukin-4 inhibits the proliferation but not the differentiation of activated human B cells in response to interleukin-2. J Exp Med 1988; 168: 1321-33.
43. DiRaimondo F, LaPushin R, Hersh EM. Synergism between alpha-Interferon and Interleukin-2-activated killer cells: In vitro studies. Acta Haematol 1987; 78: 77-83.
44. Dubinett SM, Kurnick JT, Kradin RL. Analysis of the local inflammatory response to adoptive immunotherapy with activated lymphocytes, IFN-gamma, and IL-2. FASEB J 1988; 2: 2286.
45. Dutcher JP, Creekmore S, Weiss GR, Atkins MB. A phase II study of interleukin-2 and LAK cells in patients with metastatic malignant melanoma. J Clin Oncol 1989; 7: 477-85.
46. Edwards BS, Hawkins MJ, Borden EC. Comparative in vivo and in vitro activation of human natural killer cells by two recombinant α-Interferons differing in antiviral activity. Cancer Res 1984; 44: 3135-39.
47. Edwards BS, Merritt JA, Fuhlbrigge RC, Borden EC. Low doses of interferon alpha result in more effective clinical natural killer cell activation. J Clin Invest 1985; 75: 1908-13.
48. Espevik T, Figari I, Ranges GE, Palladino MA. Transforming growth factor-β1 (TGF-β1) and recombinant human tumour necrosis factor α reciprocally regulate the generation of lymphokine-activated killer cell activity. J Immunol 1988; 140: 2312-6.
49. Farace F, Mathiot C, Brandely M, et al. Phase I trial with recombinant Interleukin-2 (rIL-2): Immune activation by rIL-2 alone or following pretreatment with recombinant Interferon-gamma. Clin Exp Immunol 1990; 82: 194-9.
50. Favrot M, Capdeville R, Combaret V, et al. Functional and phenotypic modifications induced by IL-4, as single agent or in combination with IL-2, on PBMC preactivated in vivo by alpha-Interferon + Interleukin-2 therapy. European Cytokine Network 1990; 1: 141-7.
51. Favrot M, Combaret V, Blay JY, et al. TNF alpha enhancement of NK and LAK cell functions induced by high-dose IL-2 in human peripheral blood mononuclear cells from patients pretreated with alpha IFN + IL-2. European Cytokine Network 1990; 1: 221-7.
52. Figlin RA, Belldegrun A, Moldawer N, et al. Concomitant administration of recombinant human Interleukin-2 and recombinant Interferon alfa-2A: An active outpatient regimen in metastatic renal cell carcinoma. J Clin Oncol 1992; 10: 414-21.
53. Fisher RI, Coltman CA, Doroshow JH, Paietta EL. Metastatic renal cancer treated with interleukin-2 and LAK cells. Ann Intern Med 1988; 108: 518-23.
54. Gallagher G, Wilcox F, Al-Azzawi F. Interleukin-3 and Interleukin-4 each strongly inhibit the induction and function of human LAK cells. Clin Exp Immunol 1988; 74: 166-70.
55. Gerosa F, Tommasi M, Gerosa M, Tridente G. Human recombinant interleukin-4 inhibits lymphokine-activated killer activity of sheep erythrocyte rosette-forming (E+) and -non-forming (E-) human lymphocytes. Int J Cancer 1988; 42: 902-5.
56. Gracomini P, Aguzzi A, Pestka S. Modulation by recombinant DNA leukocyte (alpha) and fibroblast (beta) interferons of the expression and shedding of HLA and tumour-associated antigens by human melanoma cells. J Immunol 1984; 133: 1649-55.
57. Hamblin J, Davies B, Sadullah S, et al. A phase II study of the treatment of metastatic malignant melanoma with a combination of dacarbazine, cis-platin, interleukin-2 (IL-2) and alfa-interferon (IFN). Eur J Cancer 1991; 27:
58. Haranaka K, Satomi N, Sakurai A. Anti-tumour activity of tumour necrosis factor against transplantable murine tumours and heterotransplanted human tumours in nude mice. Int J Cancer 1984; 34: 263-7.
59. Henney CS, Kuribayashi K, Kern DF, Gillis S. Interleukin-2 augments natural killer cell

activity. Nature 1981; 291: 335-8.
60. Herberman RB, Ortaldo JR, Mantovani A, et al. Effect of human recombinant interferon on cytotoxic activity of natural killer cells and monocytes. Cell Immunol 1982; 67: 160-7.
61. Herrmann F, Gebauer G, Lindemann A, et al. Interleukin-2 and interferon-gamma recruit different subsets of human peripheral blood monocytes to secrete interleukin-1 and tumour necrosis factor-alpha. Clin Exp Immunol 1989; 77: 97.
62. Hersh EM, Murray JL, Hong WK, et al. Phase I study of cancer therapy with recombinant interleukin-2 administered by intravenous bolus injection. Biotherapy 1989; 1: 215-26.
63. Higuchi CM, Thompson JA, Lindgren CG, et al. Induction of lymphokine-activated killer activity by interleukin 4 in human lymphocytes preactivated by interleukin 2 in vivo or in vitro. Cancer Res 1989; 49: 6487-92.
64. Hirsh M, Lipton A, Harvey H, et al. Phase I study of Interleukin-2 and Interferon alfa-2a as outpatient therapy for patients with advanced malignancy. J Clin Oncol 1990; 8: 1657-63.
65. Houghton AN, Thomson TM, Gross D, et al. Surface antigens of melanoma and melanocytes. Specificity of induction of Ia antigens by human interferon. J Exp Med 1984; 160: 255-69.
66. Huberman M, Bering H, Fallon B, et al. A phase I study of an outpatient regimen of recombinant human Interleukin-2 and alpha-2a-Interferon in patients with solid tumours. Cancer 1991; 68: 1708-13.
67. Iigo M, Sakurai M, Shimizu M, et al. Synergistic inhibition of the growth of adenocarcinoma 755 by the combination of interleukin-2 and interferon-β. Proc Jpn Acad Ser B 1986; 62: 275-8.
68. Iigo M, Sakurai M, Tamura T, et al. In vivo antitumour activity of multiple injections of recombinant Interleukin 2, alone and in combination with three different types of recombinant Interferon, on various syngeneic murine tumours. Cancer Res 48: 1988; 260-4.
69. Isaacs A, Lindenmann J: Virus interference. 1. The interferons. Proc R Soc Biol Sci 147: 258.
70. Itoh K, Shiiba K, Shimizu Y, et al. Generation of activated killer (AK) cells by recombinant Interleukin-2 (rIL 2) in collaboration with Interferon-γ (IFN-γ). J Immunol 1985; 134: 3124-9.
71. Jelinek DF, Lipsky PE. Inhibitory influence of IL-4 on human B cell responsiveness. J Immunol 1988; 141: 164-73.
72. Kanz L, Brugger W, Bross K, Mertelsmann R. Combination of cytokines: Current status and future prospects. Br J Haematol 1991; 79: 96-104.
73. Karray S, Defrance T, Merle-Beral H, Banchereau J, et al. Interleukin-4 counteracts the interleukin-2 induced proliferation of monoclonal B cells. J Exp Med 1988; 168: 85-97.
74. Kasid A, Bell GI, Director EP. Effects of transforming growth factor-β on human lymphokine-activated killer cell precursors: Autocrine inhibition of cellular proliferation and differentiation to immune killer cells. J Immunol 1988; 141: 690-8.
75. Kaufmann Y, Davidsohn J, Levanon M, et al. Lymphokine-activated killer (LAK) cells: Interferon-γ synergizes with Interleukin-2 to induce LAK cytotoxicity in homogeneous leukemic preparations. Clin Immunol Immunophathol 1991; 58: 278-88.
76. Kawakami Y, Rosenberg SA, Lotze MT. Interleukin 4 promotes the growth of tumour-infiltrating lymphocytes cytotoxic for human autologous melanoma. J Exp Med 1988; 168: 2183-91.
77. Kawakami Y, Custer MC, Rosenberg SA, Lotze MT. IL-4 regulates IL-2 induction of lymphokine-activated killer activity from human lymphocytes. J Immunol 1989; 142: 3452-61.
78. Keilholz U, Scheibenbogen C, Tilgen W, et al. Treatment of metastatic melanoma with interferon α and interleukin-2: Significant improvement with a new dosing schedule. Onkologie 1991; 14: 82.
79. Kim B, Franceschi D, Helman S, et al. Interferon inhibition of IL-2-mediated lymphocyte proliferation. Surgery 1988; 104: 390-7.
80. Kim B, Stein S, Warnaka P. Franceschi D. Enhanced in vivo therapy of pulmonary metastases with Interferon and Interleukin-2. J Surg Res 1988; 45: 66-73.
81. Kim B, Warnaka P. Enhanced survival of IFN-α augmented IL-2 therapy of pulmonary metastases: Efficacy comparable to Interleukin-2 and lymphokine activated killer cells. J Surg Res 1991; 50: 40-6.

82. Kirchner H, Körfer A, Evers P, et al. The development of neutralizing antibodies in a patient receiving subcutaneous recombinant and natural interleukin-2. Cancer 1991; 67: 1862-4.
83. Kleinermann ES, Kurzrock R, Wyatt D, et al. Activation or suppression of the tumouricidal properties of monocytes from cancer patients following treatment with human recombinant δ-interferon. Cancer Res 1986; 46: 5401-5.
84. Knop J, Taborski B, DeMaeyer-Guignard J. Selective inhibition of the generation of T suppressor cells of contact sensitivity in vitro by interferon. J Immunol 1987; 138: 3684-7.
85. Koeffler HP, Ranyard J, Yelton L. Gamma interferon induces expression of HLA-D antigen on normal and leukemic human myeloid cells. Proc Nat Acad Sci USA 1984; 81: 4080-4.
86. Kornbluth J, Hoover RG. Changes in gene expression associated with IFN-β and IL-2-induced augmentation of human natural killer cell function. J Immunol 1988; 141: 3234-40.
87. Krigel RL, Padavic-Shaller KA, Rudolph AR, et al. A phase I study of recombinant Interleukin 2 plus recombinant β-Interferon. Cancer Res 1988; 48: 3875-81.
88. Krigel RL, Padavic-Shaller KA, Rudolph AR, et al. Renal cell carcinoma: Treatment with recombinant Interleukin-2 plus Beta-Interferon. J Clin Oncol 1990; 8: 460-7.
89. Krown SE. Interferon treatment of renal cell carcinoma: Current status and future prospectives. Cancer 1987; 59: 647-51.
90. Kruit WHJ, Goey SH, Monson JRT, et al. Clinical experience with the combined use of recombinant interleukin2 (IL2) and interferon alfa-2a (IFNα) in metastatic melanoma. Br J Haematol 1991; 79: 84-6.
91. Kuribayashi K, Gillis S, Kern DE, Henney CS. Murine NK cell cultures: Effects of Interleukin-2 and Interferon on cell growth and cytotoxic reactivity. J Immunol 1981; 126: 2321-7.
92. Lauzon W, Lemaire I. Effects of biological response modifiers on lung natural killer activity. Immunopharmacol Immunotoxicol 1991; 13: 237-50.
93. Lee KH, Talpaz M, Rothberg JM, et al. Concomitant administration of recombinant human Interleukin-2 and recombinant interferon α-2A in cancer patients: A phase I study. J Clin Oncol 1989; 7: 1726-32.
94. Lee SH, Chiu H, Rinderknecht E, et al. Importance of treatment regimen of interferon as an antitumour agent. Cancer Res 1983; 43: 4172-5.
95. Legha SS. Interferons in the treatment of malignant melanoma. A review of recent trials. Cancer 1986; 57: 1675-7.
96. Legha SS, Ring S, Plager C, et al. Biochemotherapy using interleukin-2 (IL-2) + interferon alfa 2-A (IFN) in combination with cisplatin (C), vinblastine (V) and DTIC (D) in advanced melanoma. Proc AACO 1991; 10: 293.
97. Lopez Hänninen E, Körfer A, Hadam M, et al. Biological monitoring of low-dose interleukin 2 in humans: Soluble interleukin-2 receptors, cytokines, and cell surface phenotypes. Cancer Res 1991; 50: 6312-6.
98. Lynch DH, Namen AE, Miller RE. In vivo evaluation of the effects of Interleukins 2, 4 and 7 on enhancing the immunotherapeutic efficacy of anti-tumour cytotoxic T lymphocytes. Eur J Immunol 1991; 21: 2977-85.
99. Mandelli F, Tribalto M, Avvisati G. Recombinant interferon-alpha-2b as post-induction therapy for responding multiple myeloma patients. Cancer Treat Rev 1988; 15: 43-8.
100. Martinez OM, Gibbons RS, Garovoy MR, Aronson FR. IL-4 inhibits IL-2 receptor expression and IL-2-dependent proliferation of human T cells. J Immunol 1990; 144: 2211-5.
101. McBride WH, Economou JS, Nayersina R, et al. Influences of interleukins 2 and 4 on tumour necrosis factor production by murine mononuclear phagocytes. Cancer Res 1990; 50: 2949-57.
102. McIntosh JK, Mulé JJ, Merino MJ, Rosenberg SA. Synergistic antitumour effects of immunotherapy with recombinant Interleukin-2 and recombinant tumour necrosis factor-α. Cancer Res 1988; 48: 4011-7.
103. McIntosh JK, Mule JJ, Krosnick JA, Rosenberg SA. Combination cytokine immunotherapy with tumour necrosis factor α, Interleukin 2, and α-Interferon and its synergistic antitumour

effects in mice. Cancer Res 1989; 49: 1408-14.
104. Mitchell LC, Davis LS, Lipsky PE. Promotion of human T lymphocyte proliferation by IL-4. J Immunol 1989; 142: 1548-53.
105. Mittelman A, Puccio C, Ahmed T, et al. A phase II trial of Interleukin-2 by continuous infusion and Interferon by intramuscular injection in patients with renal cell carcinoma. Cancer 1991; 68: 1699-1702.
106. Mosmann TR, Bond MW, Coffman RL, et al. T cell and mast cell lines respond to B cell stimulatory factor-1. Proc Natl Acad Sci USA 1980; 83: 5654.
107. Moxey-Mims MM, Simms H, Frank MM, et al. The effects of IL-1, IL-2, and tumour necrosis factor on polymorphonuclear leukocyte Fcγ receptor-mediated phagocytosis: IL-2 down-regulates the effect of tumour necrosis factor. J Immunol 1991; 147: 1823-30.
108. Mule JJ, Smith GA, Rosenberg SA: Interleukin 4 (B cell stimulatory factor 1) can mediate the induction of lymphokin-activated killer cell activity directed against fresh tumour cells. J Exp Med 1987; 166: 792-7.
109. Mule JJ, Schwartz SL, Roberts AB, et al. Transforming growth factor-beta inhibits the in vitro generation of lymphokine-activated killer cells and cytotoxic T cells. Cancer Immunol Immunother 1988; 26: 95-102.
110. Murray JL, Pillow JK, Rosenblum MG. Differential in vitro effects of alpha recombinant interferon and gamma recombinant interferon on the expression of melanoma-associated antigens. Proc AACR 1986; 27: 313.
111. Muss HB. Interferon therapy for renal cell carcinoma. Semin Oncol 1987; 15: 36-42.
112. Narumi S, Finke JH, Hamilton TA. Interferon gamma and interleukin 2 synergize to induce selective monokine expression in murine peritoneal macrophages. J Biol Chem 1990; 265: 7036-41.
113. Nathan CF, Murray HW, Wiebe ME. Identification of interferon-gamma as the lymphokine that activates human macrophage oxidative metabolism and antimicrobial activity. J Exp Med 1983; 158: 670-89.
114. Nedwin GE, Svedersky LP, Bringman TS, et al. Effect of Interleukin 2, Interferon-δ, and mitogens on the production of tumour necrosis factors α and β. J Immunol 1985; 135: 2492-7.
115. Netaji B, Murthy S, Budd GT, et al. Phase IA/IB trial of interleukin-2 and interleukin-4 in refractory malignancy: Toxicity and immunologic changes. Proc AACR 1991; 32: 193.
116. Nishimura T, Ohta S, Sato N, et al. Combination tumour-immunotherapy with recombinant tumour necrosis factor and recombinant Interleukin-2 in mice. Int J Cancer 1987; 40: 255-61.
117. Noelle R, Krammer PH, Ohara J, et al. Increased expression of Ia antigens on resting B cells: an additional role for B-cell growth factor. Proc Nat Acad Sci USA 1984; 81: 6149-53.
118. Olencki T, Nataji B, Budd GT, et al. Phase I trial of rIL-2 and rhuIL-4 in patients with refractory malignancy: Hematologic and immunologic effects. Blood 1991; 78: 439a.
119. Ostensen ME, Thiele DL, Lipsky PE. tumour necrosis factor-α enhances cytolytic activity of human natural killer cells. J Immunol 1987; 138: 4185-91.
120. Ottesen SS, Ahrenkiel V, Kieler J. Recombinant human interferon-γ exerts an antiproliferative effects and modulates the expression of human leukocyte antigens A, B, C, and DR. Cancer Immunol Immunother 1990; 31: 93-8.
121. Owen-Schaub LB, Gutterman JU, Grimm EA. Synergy of tumour necrosis factor and Interleukin 2 in the activation of human cytotoxic lymphocytes: Effect of tumour necrosis factor α and Interleukin 2 in the generation of human lymphokine-activated killer cell cytotoxicity. Cancer Res 1988; 48: 788-92.
122. Pace JL, Russell SW, Torres BA, et al. Recombinant mouse γ-interferon induces the priming step in macrophage activation for tumour cell killing. J Immunol 1983; 130: 2011-3.
123. Palladino MA, Czarniecki CW, Chiu HH, et al. Regulation of cytokine production and class II antigen expression by transforming growth factor-β. J Cell Biochem 1987; (Suppl 11A): 10.
124. Paolozzi F, Zamkoff K, Doyle M, et al. Phase I trial of recombinant interleukin-2 and recombinant beta-interferon in refractory neoplastic diseases. J Biol Response Mod 1989; 8: 122-39.

125. Pichert G, Jost LM, Fierz W, Stahel RA. Clinical and immune modulatory effects of alternative weekly Interleukin-2 and Interferon alfa-2a in patients with advanced renal cell carcinoma and melanoma. Br J Cancer 1991; 63: 287-92.
126. Puri RK, Travis WD, Rosenberg SA. In vivo administration of Interferon α and Interleukin 2 induces proliferation of lymphoid cells in the organs of mice. Cancer Res 1990; 50: 5543-50.
127. Puri RK, Leland P. In vivo treatment with Interferon causes augmentation of IL-2 induced lymphokine-activated killer cells in the organs of mice. Clin Exp Immunol 1991; 85: 317-25.
128. Quesada JR, Rios A, Swanson D. Antitumour activity of recombinant-derived interferon alpha in metastatic renal cell carcinoma. J Clin Oncol 1985; 3: 1522-28.
129. Quesada JR, Alexanian R, Hawkins M, et al. Treatment of multiple myeloma with recombinant alpha-interferon. Blood 1986; 67: 275-8.
130. Quesada JR, Hersh EM, Manning J. Treatment of hairy-cell leukemia with recombinant alpha interferon. Blood 1986; 68: 493-7.
131. Ranges GE, Figari IS, Espevik T, Palladino MA. Inhibition of cytotoxic T cell development by transforming growth factor and reversal by recombinant tumour necrosis factor. J Exp Med 1987; 166: 991-8.
132. Rawlinson L, Dalton BJ, Rogers K, Rees RC. The influence of interferon, alpha and gamma, singly or in combination on human natural cell mediated cytotoxicity. Biosci Rep 1988; 9: 459-56.
133. Redman BG, Flaherty L, Chou TH, et al. A phase I trial of recombinant Interleukin-2 combined with recombinant Interferon-gamma in patients with cancer. J Clin Oncol 1990; 8: 1269-76.
134. Richards JM: Sequential chemo-immunotherapy for metastatic melanoma. Semin Oncol 1991; 18: 91-95.
135. Rook AH, Kehrl JH, Wakefield LM, et al. Effects of transforming growth factor β on the functions of natural killer cells: Depressed cytolytic activity and blunting of Interferon responsiveness. J Immunol 1986; 136: 3916-20.
136. Rosenberg SA, Lotze MT, Chang AE, et al. A progress report on the treatment of 157 patients with advanced cancer using lymphokine-activated killer cells and interleukin-2 or high-dose interleukin-2 alone. N Engl J Med 1987; 316: 889-97.
137. Rosenberg SA, Schwarz SL, Spiess PJ. Combination immunotherapy for cancer: Synergistic antitumour interactions of Interleukin-2, alfa Interferon, and tumour-infiltrating lymphocytes. J Natl Cancer Inst 1988; 80: 1393-7.
138. Rosenberg SA, Lotze MT, Yang JC, et al. Experience with the use of high-dose Interleukin-2 in the treatment of 652 cancer patients. Ann Surg 1989; 210: 474-85.
139. Rosenberg SA, Lotze MT, Yang JC, et al. Combination therapy with Interleukin-2 and alpha-Interferon for the treatment of patients with advanced cancer. J Clin Oncol 1989; 7: 1863-74.
140. Schipper H, Clinch J, McMurray A, Levitt M. Measuring the quality of life of cancer patients: the functional living index - cancer: development and validation. J Clin Oncol 1984; 2: 472-83.
141. Silagi S, Dutkowski R, Schaefer A. Eradication of mouse melanoma by combined treatment with recombinant human Interleukin 2 and recombinant murine Interferon-gamma. Int J Cancer 1988; 41: 315-22.
142. Sone S, Utsugi T, Nii A, Ogura T. Differential effects of recombinant Interferons α, β, and γ on induction of human lymphokine (IL-2)-activated killer activity. J Natl Cancer Inst 1988; 80: 425-31.
143. Sosman JA, Kohler PC, Hank JA, Sondel PM. Repetitive weekly cycles of interleukin-2. Clinical and immunologic effects of dose, schedule, and addition of indomethacin. J Natl Cancer Inst 1988; 80: 1451-61.
144. Spits H, Yssel H, Takebe Y, et al. Recombinant Interleukin 4 promotes the growth of human T cells. J Immunol 1987; 139: 1142-7.
145. Spits H, Yssel H, Paliard X, et al. IL-4 inhibits IL-2-mediated induction of human lymphokine-activated killer cells, but not the generation of antigen-specific cytotoxic T

lymphocytes in mixed leukocyte cultures. J Immunol 1988; 141: 29-36.

146. Splawski JB, Jelinek DF, Lipsky PE. Immunomodulatory role of IL-4 on the secretion of Ig by human B cells. J Immunol 1986; 142: 1569-75.
147. Sporn MB, Robert AB, Wakefield LM, Assoian RK. Transforming growth factor-β: biological function and chemical structure. Science 1986; 233: 532-4.
148. Suzuki R, Suzuki S, Ebina N, Kumagai K. Suppression of alloimmune cytotoxic T lymphocyte (CTL) generation by depletion of NK cells and restoration by Interferon and/or Interleukin 2. J Immunol 1985; 134: 2139-48.
149. Svedersky LP, Shepard HM, Spencer SA, et al. Augmentation of human natural cell-mediated cytotoxicity by recombinant human interleukin-2. J Immunol 1984; 133: 714-8.
150. Svedersky LP, Nedwin GE, Goeddel DV, et al. Interferon-γ enhances induction of lymphotoxin in recombinant Interleukin 2-stimulated peripheral blood mononuclear cells. J Immunol 1985; 134: 1604-8.
151. Sznol M Janik JE, Sharfman WH, et al. A phase Ia/Ib study of subcutaneously (SQ) administered interleukin-2 (IL-2) in combination with interferon-alfa 2a (IFN). Proc AACO 1991; 10: 209.
152. Talpaz M, Kantarjian HM, McCreedie K. Hematologic remission and cytogenetic improvement induced by recombinant human interferon alpha A in chronic myelogenous leukemia. N Engl J Med 1986; 314: 1065-9.
153. Tamura T. Sasaki Y, Shinkai T, et al. Phase I study of combination therapy with Interleukin 2 and β-Interferon in patients with advanced malignancy. Cancer Res. 1989; 49: 730-5.
154. Thompson JA, Lee DJ, Lindgren CG, et al. Influence of dose and duration of interleukin-2 on toxicity and immunomodulation. J Clin Oncol 1988; 6: 669-78.
155. Tokuda Y, Ebina N, Golub SH. The inhibitory effect of human Interferon alpha on the generation of lymphokine- activated killer activity. Cancer Immunol Immunother 1989; 30: 205-12.
156. Toledano M, Mathiot C, Michon J, et al. Interferon-γ and interleukin-2 in the generation of lymphokine-activated killer cell cytotoxicity. Cancer Immunol Immunother 1989; 30: 57-62.
157. Treismann J, Higuchi CM, Thompson JA, et al. Enhancement by Interleukin 4 of Interleukin 2- or antibody-induced proliferation of lymphocytes from Interleukin 2-treated cancer patients. Cancer Res 1990; 50: 1160-4.
158. Truitt GA, Stern LL, Bontempo J. Recombinant human Interleukin-2 (IL-2), alone and in combination with Interferon alpha, is a potent antitumour agent against colon 38 and Lewis lung carcinomas in mice. Proc AACR 1987; 28: 369.
159. Vaage J. Peri-tumour interleukin-2 causes systemic therapeutic effect via interferon-γ induction. Int J Cancer 1991; 49: 598-600.
160. VanDeGriend RJ, Ronteltap CPM, Gravekamp C, et al. Interferon-β and recombinant interleukin-2 can both enhance, but by different pathways, the nonspecific cytolytic potential of T3-negative natural killer cell-derived clones rather than that of T3-positive clones. J Immunol 1986; 136: 1700-7.
161. Wahl SM, Hunt DA, Wong HL, et al. Transforming growth factor-β is a potent immunosuppressive agent that inhibits IL-1-dependent lymphocyte proliferation. J Immunol 1988; 40: 3026-32.
162. Wan YJ, Orrison BM, Lieberman R. Induction of major histocompatibility class I antigens by interferons in undifferentiated F9 cells. J Cell Physiol 1987; 130: 276-83.
163. Weiner LM, Padavic-Shaller K, Kitson J, et al. Phase I evaluation of combination therapy with interleukin 2 and γ-interferon. Cancer Res 1991; 51: 3910-8.
164. Weiss GR, Margolin KA, Aronson FR, et al. A randomized phase II trial of continuous infusion interleukin-2 or bolus injection interleukin-2 plus lymphokine-activated killer cells for advanced renal cell carcinoma. J Clin Oncol 1992; 10: 275-81.
165. West WH, Tauer KW, Yannelli JR, et al. Constant-infusion recombinant interleukin-2 in adoptive immunotherapy of advanced cancer. N Engl J Med 1987; 316: 898-905.
166. West WH. Clinical application of continuous infusion of recombinant Interleukin-2. Eur J

Cancer Clin Oncol 1989; 25: 11-15.

167. Widmer MB, Acres BR, Sassenfeld HM, Grabstein KH. Regulation of cytolytic cell populations from human peripheral blood by B cell stimulatory factor 1 (Interleukin 4). J Exp Med 1987; 166: 1447-55.
168. Winkelhake JI, Stampfl S, Zimmerman RJ. Synergistic effects of combination therapy with human recombinant interleukin 2 and tumour necrosis factor in murine tumour models. Cancer Res 1987; 47: 3948-53.
169. Yang SC, Owen-Schaub LB, Grimm EA, Roth JA. Induction of lymphokine-activated killer cytotoxicity with interleukin-2 and tumour necrosis factor-α against primary lung cancer targets. Cancer Immunol Immunother 1989; 29: 193-108.
170. Yang SC, Grimm EA, Parkinson DR, et al. Clinical and immunomodulatory effects of combination immunotherapy with low-dose interleukin 2 and tumour necrosis factor α in patients with advanced non-small cell lung cancer: A phase I trial. Cancer Res 1991; 51: 3669-76.
171. Zamkoff K, Newman N, Paolozzi F, et al. A phase I study of recombinant interleukin-2 and recombinant beta interferon in patients with advanced malignancy. Proc AACR 1987; 6: 242.

10. Future prospects for Interleukin-2 therapy

CHRISTOPHER R. FRANKS and PETER A. PALMER

1. Introduction

The clinical development of Interleukin-2 has been possible because the advent of biotechnology has resulted in the availability of unrestricted quantities of recombinant Interleukin-2 (rIL-2). Since there is little or no precedence, the initial investigational criteria used were those established for the evaluation of conventional cancer drugs [1]; that is the identification and subsequent administration of the maximum tolerated dose, and the assessment of efficacy based on objective response rate. However, since rIL-2 is an immune stimulant, and has no direct action as an anti-tumour agent [2, 3], it does not make sense to evaluate the compound using standard oncological criteria. A more global concept of efficacy (objective response, quality of life, and survival) would seem to be more relevant [4].

In retrospect, the positioning of rIL-2 as an anti-cancer agent may have retarded to some degree the development of its true potential. There are a number of non-cancer indications in which rIL-2 could have a therapeutic role. Since the compound is pleiotropic [5, 6], it has a variety of functions in vivo (discussed in other chapters), in addition to being a growth factor for T-cells. Some of these may contribute to therapeutic effects, and some to the toxicity of the compound. The dose response for each of these may be different.

There is therefore unlikely to be a single optimum treatment schedule, but an optimal dose for a particular schedule, resulting in treatment intensities which achieve comparable efficacies [7]. In the circumstances, the search for *the* optimal dose and schedule may be ill-founded.

The effective use of immunotherapy in medicine therefore requires a pragmatic approach. By evaluating these new therapeutic concepts in context, the true potential of an innovative compound like IL-2 may be realised.

J. Wagstaff (ed.), The Role of Interleukin-2 in the Treatment of Cancer Patients, 169-185.

2. Use of rIL-2 in the treatment of bacterial and iatrogenic immune-suppression

There are a wide variety of clinical settings in which immune-suppressed states occur, either as a result of disease, or as a result of treatment. The role for IL-2-based therapy in the above settings may be particularly relevant.

2.1. Bacteria-induced immune-suppression

A number of experimental models have shown that some bacteria can cause defective endogenous IL-2 production [6]. Several workers have found that high doses of mycobacterium bovis BCG (M Bovis), injected into rodents, results in T-cell unresponsiveness [8, 9]. Colizzi [10] reported that this T-cell unresponsiveness can be reversed, using very low doses of rIL-2. Although, a lot more basic work is necessary before it is possible to determine whether rIL-2 can play a positive role in the management of similar disease states in man, it is not unreasonable to speculate that the administration of systemic rIL-2 may be beneficial where in vivo IL-2 production is suppressed.

2.2. Treatment-induced immune-suppression

Surprisingly, very little research has occurred using rIL-2 in settings where treatment results in immune-suppression. It has long been known that major surgery induces a marked reduction in cellular immunity, both in animals and in man [11–14]. The clinical repercussions, in patients with cancer, may therefore be significant, since surgical intervention may adversely alter the post-surgical progression of an otherwise surgically curable malignancy [15].

Attempts to use non-specific immune-modulators, such as Levamisole [16] have proved to be very disappointing. A profound lymphocytopenia is a common finding in patients during the post-surgical period. In the absence of heterologous transfusions, this may persist for up to 10 days. A correlation has been reported between the degree of lymphocytopenia and the occurrence of distant metastases in patients with colorectal cancer [17]. Although it may be simplistic to suggest that abrogation of the lymphocytopenia will have a positive impact on the subsequent development of metastases, Carp et al. [18] have recently reported animal studies, which demonstrate that the concept is a reality in vivo. Recombinant IL-2 was administered three days before and three days following laparotomy in an experimental mouse model. All the mice were injected with murine pancreatic adenocarcinoma, and were randomised to receive no further treatment, laparotomy, or laparotomy plus perioperative rIL-2 (10^6 IU/day). The administration of rIL-2 not only led to a reduction in the potential of the tumour to metastasize to the lung, but there was also a reversal of the surgically-induced immune suppression, as measured by the responsiveness of splenic lymphocytes to mitogen in vitro.

In a recent pilot study, Brivio et al. [19] have evaluated a similar concept in man. Recombinant IL-2 was administered subcutaneously for three days prior to surgery, using a dose of 18 × 10^6 IU/m^2. All five patients had colon cancer. When the patients were compared with control patients, undergoing surgery for the same tumour, the number of lymphocytes, T lymphocytes, NK cells, and CD-25+ cells were significantly higher in the patients receiving rIL-2. In addition, there were no surgical or medical complications during the post-operative period, and the toxicity profile was found to be very acceptable. These observations are now being critically evaluated in a controlled clinical trials programme.

3. Regional administration

Roth et al. [20] and Bubenik [21] have both proposed theoretical rationales for using rIL-2 as regional therapy in certain tumour types. The toxicity of systemic treatment, the potential to deliver high concentrations of drug at the tumour site, and the knowledge that IL-2 is a hormone with a range of action measured in microns (under normal physiological conditions in vivo), are obvious stimuli for further research. This is of particular interest in malignancies, where tumour invasion may be regional, or confined to one organ site or body cavity, but where curative surgery and/or radiotherapy is not possible [20].

3.1. Intra-pleural therapy

In a recent phase I study, in patients with malignant pleural mesothelioma, Eggermont [22] reported very promising anti-tumour activity, using non-toxic doses of rIL-2, given by continuous infusion for 14 days, via an intra-pleural portacath. Four partial responders were recorded in 10 patients, treated at daily doses of 30 × 10^3 IU to 30 × 10^5 IU. No responses were seen in 7 patients treated at higher doses. These data suggest that intra-pleural administration of rIL-2 can result in meaningful anti-tumour activity at non-toxic doses. However, since the patient population is rather small, additional studies should be carried out to confirm these interesting findings. Patients with malignant pleural effusions, due to other malignancies apart from mesothelioma, should also be included in such a trial.

3.2. Intra-peritoneal therapy

Although intra-peritoneal (i.p.) administration of rIL-2, in patients with ovarian cancer, seems to be a reasonable target indication, the data generated to date in fact suggest that this is contra-indicated, because of the development of intra-peritoneal fibrosis [23, 24]. These problems have somewhat discouraged further investigation. In the circumstances, this therapeutic approach, using i.p. rIL-2, may not be actively pursued in the future.

3.3. Intra-vesical therapy

Another indication, suitable for investigation of local cytokine therapy, is non-metastatic transitional cell carcinoma of the bladder. There have been some encouraging results, using intra-lesional injections of partially purified native IL-2 [25]. Three, of ten patients with invasive bladder cancer, achieved a complete response. Huland et al. [26] have also reported anti-tumour activity, using continuous intra-vesical rIL-2 infusion. Velotti et al. [27] investigated the effects of continuous intra-arterial infusion (using the internal iliac artery), in patients with superficial transitional cell cancer of the bladder. Complete responses were noted in three patients, using a daily dose of 18×10^4 IU. No responses were seen at lower or higher doses.

Although the above approaches are interesting from an experimental standpoint, the techniques are too cumbersome to be used as a routine treatment in hospital practice, and are therefore unlikely to be developed further.

Intravesical immuno-therapy with BCG, or chemotherapy using thiotepa, mitomycin or doxorubicin, is currently considered as the treatment of choice for the management of non-metastatic transitional cell tumours of the bladder. The side effects of conventional treatment, the fact that patients, who respond to BCG, appear to have detectable levels of IL-2 in the urine, following BCG treatment [28], and the responses noted in the rIL-2 pilot studies, all provide a reasonable rationale for further evaluating rIL-2 as a potential treatment option.

In 1991, Tubaro et al. [29] reported the results of a phase Ib study. Twelve patients, with Ta-T1, G1-2, NO, MO primary or recurrent transitional cell carcinoma of the bladder, received 10 daily intravesical instillations of rIL-2. Additional instillations were administered one month following clinical response evaluation and transurethral resection of tumour. The latter cytokine treatment was then repeated at 4 monthly intervals for one year. Partial responses were observed in 2 patients. No relapses were seen at the median of 6.5 months (range 1 to 14 months). These preliminary data have been a stimulus for more studies using the above treatment concepts, although alternative therapeutic approaches may be to combine rIL-2 and BCG, or to test combinations of rIL-2 and other cytokines and/or chemotherapy.

3.4. Peri-tumour therapy

Several workers [21, 30–32] have demonstrated that local repetitive peri-tumoral injections of rIL-2 (given subcutaneously in the area of the lymph nodes draining tumour) can inhibit the growth of subcutaneously transplanted 3-methylcolantrene (MC) induced sarcomas in syngenic mice. However, the results should be interpreted with caution, since the experimental setting is one of an immunogenic tumour, which may not be of relevance in man. Nevertheless, the studies do demonstrate that rIL-2 is active, if given directly into an immunogenic tumour [6]. If strategies can be developed to assist the immune system of the host to actively recognise poorly immunogenic tumours, the local administration of rIL-2, or combinations of cytokines, may not only lead to rejection of tumour, but, more significantly, to a sustained immunological memory thus preventing relapse.

The work of Forni et al. [33] falls into the above context. Using a low immunogenic MC-induced sarcoma tumour (CE-2), local IL-2 injections, at very low doses (10 Units/day for 10 days), resulted in the rejection of the CE-2 tumour in only 25% of mice. When tumour cells were injected, together with nylon wool adherent spleen lymphocytes (TB-Ly), there was no apparent inhibition of tumour. In contrast, when the mice were challenged with tumour, together with TB-Ly and local very low dose IL-2 for 10 days, an almost complete inhibition of tumour was observed, and 96% survival. This combined approach, designated LATI (Lymphokine Activated Tumour Inhibition), should not be confused with the adoptive transfer of lymphokine activated lymphoid cells. Analysis of the possible mechanisms of LATI, demonstrate that transferred TB-Ly cells are not directly involved in tumour cell killing, but in the recruitment and stimulation of host effector T-lymphocytes, NK cells, monocytes, and eosinophils, ultimately leading to tumour destruction. Moreover, irradiated TB-Ly cells can still achieve LATI, suggesting that an IL-2 dependent clonal expansion of transferred lymphoid cells is not required. Tumour destruction was inhibited by sub-lethal total body irradiation, suggesting that the systemic immune response of the host is important in the LATI phenomenon. The most provocative finding is that mice, surviving the original tumour challenge due to LATI, were specifically protected against a subsequent challenge with CE-2 tumour cells, but not to a challenge with other tumour types. This provides strong evidence of a tumour-specific memory, elicited by the LATI phenomenon.

These pre-clinical findings have stimulated pilot studies in patients with recurrent squamous cell carcinoma of the head and neck [34–37]. Very low doses of rIL-2 were given perilymphatically, and peritumorally. Short-lived objective responses were seen in 6 of 10 patients treated in the first study [34], but no responses were seen in the second study [35]. This may be due to patient selection criteria, particularly the size of the tumour, its location, and the presence or absence of contra-lateral or bi-lateral cervical lymph nodes. Musiani et al. [37] reported on the histological evaluation of tumour and lymph nodes recovered at surgery, following pre-operative perilymphatic treatment with low dose rIL-2. The picture was one of degenerating neoplastic cells, massively surrounded by lymphocytes, large granular lymphocytes, and eosinophils. These findings are reminiscent of the findings in the murine models discussed above. However, tumour regression was short-lived, indicating that a sustained immunological memory was not achieved. At this point in time, it is unclear whether the difference between the animal and human studies is species-specific, and/or due to immune-suppression present in man. What is clear is that the pre-clinical findings need further investigation, and, through a better understanding of the complex interactions between host and tumour, novel treatment modalities may be identified in the future.

4. Use of rIL-2 in the treatment of viral infectious diseases

Immunotherapy is most logicial in situations where the immune system requires support. This may be true for cancer, but may also be true in viral infectious diseases. In contrast to the vast literature on the experimental use of rIL-2 in cancer, much less research has been done to investigate the potential of IL-2-based therapy in viral disease settings. Although there may be major differences between the two patient populations, the common denominator is that the immune system requires boosting to a sufficient level to overcome host tolerance.

4.1. HIV

Patients with HIV were amongst the first to be treated with IL-2, when sufficient quantities became available for clinical testing. HIV infects lymphocytes, particularly CD4 (helper-inducer) cells, resulting in both qualitative and quantitative deficits. Production and responsiveness to IL-2 is decreased in the peripheral blood of HIV positive patients. In vitro studies have shown that IL-2 has a potential to correct some of these deficits [38, 39].

The first human studies used purified IL-2 from the Jurkat T-cell line, and was given i.v. at low doses [40, 41], or subcutaneously [42]. No meaningful clinical benefits were seen. Higher doses, for prolonged periods, resulted in some anecdotal clinical benefits in a minority of patients [43], but durable immune enhancement was not found. In addition, there was some concern that IL-2 could stimulate viral replication [44].

Recently, rIL-2 has been combined with Zidovudine (AZT) in the treatment of patients with a more favourable prognosis [45]. The results have been encouraging. There has been no evidence of enhanced viral replication, and durable increases in CD4 counts have been noted, lasting more than 10 months following cessation of therapy. Such findings warrant further investigation. The relevant trials have now been activated.

Although only relatively few patients with Kaposi's sarcoma have been treated with rIL-2 to date [46](using a continuous infusion schedule), no positive effect has been noted, apart from the absence of treatment-related toxicity. However, in HIV-associated lymphomas, 2 of 4 pretreated patients have achieved a good partial response, and 2 stable disease, using a combination of AZT and rIL-2 [47]. At the end of rIL-2 therapy, all patients were P-24 negative. At 2–3 months follow-up, P-24 became positive in 2 patients, and both demonstrated increased HIV growth in vitro. Despite these findings, there was no progression of lymphoma or manifestation of AIDS in either patient. Following treatment, CD4 increased from a mean of 104/μL (range 43–220/μL) to 220/μL (range 90–266/μL). In addition, both LAK and NK activity showed small increases from 69% to 81% and 73% to 75% respectively. This impact of rIL-2 on HIV-associated lymphomas is an interesting finding and is being studied further.

4.2. Hepatitis B

Factors determining the outcome of infection with hepatitis B virus (HBV) are not fully understood. Patients, who do not clear the virus after the first infection, become chronic HBsAg carriers, and often develop chronic active hepatitis B.

Based on the hypothesis, that development of the chronic state is a result of incompetence of the immune system, a number of small studies have been performed, using native Interleukin-2 (nIL-2) or rIL-2. Most of the studies have been carried out in Japan [48–51]. The results should be interpreted with caution, since the epidemiology of HBV, and the response to antiviral therapy (e.g. IFN-alpha) in the Orient, appears to be markedly different from that seen in the West [52]. In addition, it is difficult to identify what dose of IL-2 was administered. From the literature, the following observations emerge: low doses of rIL-2, in the range of 600,000 IU, given over 1 week, are less effective than the same dose over longer periods of time (28 days). Toxicity is mainly limited to mild flu-like symptoms, and is less problematic than IFN-alpha. Although occasional patients seroconvert to anti-HBeAg, this remains within the range of spontaneous seroconversion (0–30%). During rIL-2 therapy, a marked decrease in HBV specific DNA polymerase activity is seen, but is usually only noted whilst treatment is ongoing.

Surprisingly, the initial trials in the West did not consider these results within the context of the trial design. For example, a pilot study was activated and subsequently abandoned after only 4 patients had been treated, due to unacceptable toxicity [53]. Patients received 24×10^6 IU/m^2 IL-2, 3 times a week for 12 weeks. The rationale for using this dose and schedule is unclear, and the toxicity could have been anticipated. The schedule seems to have been inspired by clinical trials in the oncological setting, which is completely inappropriate.

In a phase I study, reported by Vogel et al. [54], using nIL-2 given s.c., an attempt was made to identify an optimal biological dose, based on the induction of secondary cytokines and cytokine-dependent serum components (including neopterin and soluble IL-2 receptor). No evidence of anti-viral activity was seen however.

Only one small pilot study has been reported, using prolonged rIL-2 administration plus alpha-IFN [55]. The anti-viral activity of IFN is well-documented, with approximately 30% of patients responding by seroconversion. It was postulated that the combination with rIL-2 would increase the response rate because of the differential activity of rIL-2 and IFN. In the study, 4 out of 8 patients responded by seroconversion. Based on these findings, a multi-centre randomised trial is in progress in Europe, but more studies will be needed to further investigate whether prolonged rIL-2 therapy alone, or in combination with anti-viral agents, has a role in the treatment of patients with chronic hepatitis B.

5. rIL-2 as an adjuvant to vaccination

5.1. Infectious diseases

Pre-clinical studies have demonstrated a potential for the use of rIL-2 as an adjuvant to vaccination. In a swine model, Anderson et al. [56] found enhanced protection against Haemophilus pleuropneumonia, when rIL-2 was given systemically during, and 4 days following, vaccination. There was, however, no correlation between protection and the development of serum antibodies to the pathogen. Similar findings have been reported by Nunberg et al. [57] in a mouse rabies vaccination model. As above, there was no evidence of an increased antibody titer to rabies. Taken together, these observations suggest that cellular immunity is responsible for the potentiating effects in these particular models. This contrasts to other reports, where IL-2 seemed to act as a successful adjuvant, leading to enhanced specific antibody production, when administered locally mixed with vaccine [58]. Therefore, IL-2 may not be playing a single role, when it is used as an adjuvant.

These experiments should be taken into consideration when planning clinical trials. If an inability to achieve successful vaccination is due to a defect in cellular immunity, then the use of systemic IL-2 as an adjuvant may be appropriate. On the other other hand, if the objective is to increase the potency of vaccination, in settings where antibody production is defective, then local administration may be the first choice for investigation.

The only published clinical work in this field has been reported by Meuer et al. [59]. Uraemic patients, on long-term haemodialysis, are frequently non-responsive to vaccination with hepatitis B vaccine [60]. It is postulated that this is due to a defect in monocyte function, and, as a consequence, T-lymphocytes do not receive the signal(s) required for the production of IL-2 following antigen contact [59]. This antigen-induced activation of T-cells is necessary in order to generate the appropriate cascade, which then leads to specific antibody production [61]. Administration of a single low dose of intramuscular (i.m.) nIL-2 (75,000 IU) 4 hours after i.m. vaccination with HB vaccine (HBVax), close to the HBVax site, resulted in 6 out of 8 previously non-responsive patients seroconverting. This correlated with an enhanced in vitro response of lymphocytes to IL-2 at base-line [60]. Such findings clearly warrant further rationally designed research.

5.2. Cancer

Immune modulation has been investigated in cancer for a number of years [62–64], particularly in patients with malignant melanoma [65, 66], since this tumour has always been considered to be relatively immunogenic. Response rates with various immune modulators appear to be in the range of 20%, with reported long-term remissions and clinically significant disease stabilisation [67].

Mitchell et al. [68] have taken the concept further, using a mixture of mechanical lysates (homogenates) of 2 melanoma cell-lines, which are injected together with an adjuvant Detox. Twenty-two patients were studied in a phase I trial. Thirteen of the 22 patients had evidence of successful immunisation. An increase in antibody titer against melanoma-associated antigens, measured by enzyme immuno-assay, was found in 5 of 22 patients, and a change in delayed hyper-sensitivity against the melanoma lysate in 3 patients. Responders were found at all dose levels, without an obvious dose response. Peripheral blood cytolytic lymphocyte precursors appeared to be more reactive against melanoma cells in 12 patients. These were atypical T-cells, which recognised melanoma-associated antigens on several allogeneic lines, without apparent major histo-compatibility complex restriction. Five of 17 patients, with measurable lesions, achieved a remission, 2 of which were complete responses, and 3 partial responses, with an additional 3 minor responses. The patients with an increase in cytolytic lymphocyte precursors were the same patients who went into clinical remission. None of the 7 patients, lacking an increase in cytotoxic lymphocytes, had a clinical response. Clearly, the use of IL-2, as an adjuvant in this scenario, may well contribute to a greater number of responding patients.

In a recent paper, Mitchell et al. [69] reported that studies would be initiated in which rIL-2 was to be combined with the lysate, together with cyclophosphamide. The rationale is to try and enhance the level of cytotoxic lymphocytes stimulated by the lysate, while at the same time reducing the level of tumour-specific T suppressor cells by cyclosphosamide. Although the latter cells are somewhat difficult to measure precisely in humans, the assumption is made that they may potentially interfere with the ability to achieve successful immunisation. In addition to rIL-2, other cytokines, including IL-1, may potentially be combined with the lysate, since IL-1 has been found to be active in increasing immunity to renal cell carcinoma in mice [69].

6. Gene therapy

The identification in 1980 of lymphokine activated killer cells (LAK) by Rosenberg and colleagues [70, 71], and their use in patients [72, 73) has subsequently led to a search for immune cells which can improve therapeutic effectiveness when used in adoptive therapy. In 1986, Rosenberg et al. [74]

reported on their findings of a specific class of T-lymphocytes with unusual anti-tumour activity, which they called tumour infiltrating lymphocytes (TIL). These cells infiltrate into growing tumours, and can be grown by culturing in IL-2 single cell suspensions obtained from tumours [75].

Extensive in vivo studies have demonstrated that TIL are 50–100 times more effective in treating established lung and liver metastases in experimental models, when compared with LAK cells [74]. What is particularly interesting about TIL is that the cells recognise unique antigens on the tumours of some patients with melanoma, breast cancer, colon cancer, and lymphomas [76]. Studies with labelled TIL clearly demonstrate that TIL accumulates in tumours [77, 78]. It has been postulated, that, using gene transfer techniques, new properties can be introduced into TIL to enhance existing functions, or to generate a new kind of lymphocyte that does not exist in man. Together with colleagues from the National Heart, Lung and Blood Institute, and the National Cancer Institute, Rosenberg has initiated a study using genetically modified TIL [79].

The gene coding for neomycin phosphotransferase has been inserted into TIL cells. This provides the cells with a bacterial enzyme marker which is resistant to the antibiotic neomycin. It is therefore possible to study the long-term distribution and survival of the modified cells in humans. This is important, since retroviral-mediated gene transduction was used to introduce the neomycin gene into TIL. Clearly, there are potential dangers, because there is a possibility that replication-competent virus might be produced by recombination of vector sequences with viral coding sequences present in the packaging cell line. Extreme care was taken to minimise the possibility of helper virus generation [80, 81].

In May 1989, the first patient received gene modified TIL cells. The results in 5 patients were reported in 1990 [82]. All had widespread metastatic melanoma. Two of the 5 patients achieved objective responses. The studies demonstrated that retroviral mediated gene transduction could be safely used to genetically modify cells.

These initial gene transfer studies suggested that it might be possible to design TIL with increased therapeutic activity. The first of these 'designer' TIL cells carry the gene for Tumour Necrosis Factor (TNF), since TNF is a very effective therapeutic agent in rodents [83–86]. Unfortunately, similar activity has not been seen in man, because escalating doses of TNF result in severe toxicity [87–89]. By designing a new cell (TNF-TIL), it is postulated that it will be possible to target tumours with high doses of TNF, without causing general toxicity.

In January 1991, the first 2 patients, with metastatic melanoma, were treated with the TNF gene modified TIL [79]. No side effects were seen due to TNF-TIL, and no efficacy data are currently available.

More recently, Rosenberg and colleagues [79] have initiated studies using genetically modified cancer cells, the intention being to increase their immunogenicity, by the introduction of cytokine genes into the tumour cells

[90–93]. These immune manipulations are at a very early stage, but, as increased knowledge accrues about the nature of the immune response to human tumours, more sophisticated approaches should be possible. It is encouraging that some bulky human tumours appear to be responsive to immunological manoeuvres. Clearly, it is mandatory that the further development of this exciting technology results in an effective, safe, and practical treatment, which can be made available to the majority of patients.

7. Risk/benefit ratio

In the assessment of risk/benefit ratio, rIL-2 must be evaluated in context. Since rIL-2 is an immune-modulator, and has no specific anti-tumour effect, it seems inappropriate to evaluate efficacy primarily in terms of objective response (the standard oncological criteria), although it is understandable why this has occurred, since the first clinical studies with rIL-2 were carried out in patients with cancer [72]. In a recent review of 327 patients with renal cell cancer, treated with a continuous infusion rIL-2 schedule, a highly significant survival advantage was observed for patients receiving rIL-2 ($p < .0001$), when compared to the renal cell cancer database from the Eastern Cooperative Oncology Group [94]. The patients were sub-divided into risk categories, which were based on the assessment of quality of life (performance status), metastatic status, and the interval from diagnosis to treatment. Not only did this facilitate comparison of patient with patient, but the incorporation of these factors into a more global analysis of efficacy seems to be more compatible with the way in which biologicals achieve their effect (by mobilising host defense mechanisms). The preoccupation with objective response, as the criteria of efficacy in biotherapy does not make sense, and would seem to have little relevance when treating patients with drugs like IL-2, apart from providing an early indication of potential activity in clinical trials.

A great deal has also been written about the adverse events following treatment with rIL-2. Although there is clear evidence that toxicity is dose and schedule dependent [95], it is not necessary to generate severe toxicity (by giving high doses of rIL-2) in order to achieve an optimal objective response [96–98], contrary to some of the observations made in the scientific press [99]. Reduction of the rIL-2 dose, and/or modification of the schedule, results in treatment programmes which remain effective, but have the added advantage that they are more acceptable, both to the patient and to the physician, since treatment-induced morbidity is reduced significantly [96–98]. In the circumstances, it remains to be seen whether there is a need for alternative methods of abrogating rIL-2-induced toxicity, such as the use of inhibitors of nitric oxide generation [100], leukocyte endothelial adhesion [101], and neuro-hormones [102], all of which impact on the vascular leak syndrome, the major dose limiting side effect of high dose rIL-2.

If the advantages, resulting from IL-2 therapy, are critically compared to the potential disadvantages, the risk/benefit ratio appears to be in favour of the patient, the basic assumption being made, of course, that efficacy is being seen. Apart from the fact that treatment is usually limited (median 2 courses (range 1 to 5)), which has an impact on drug-induced side-effects, many patients now receive outpatient therapy, where morbidity is significantly reduced.

8. Conclusions

The introduction of rIL-2 into clinical medicine in the mid 80's has been a relatively quiet revolution. Although an enormous amount of research has been carried out throughout the world, there are still many unknowns. Nevertheless, great progress has been made.

It is no longer necessary to treat patients in the protected environment of the intensive care unit, since therapy can now be given safely at home. Objective responses, and even survival (in renal cell cancer, for example), appear to be very similar regardless of the schedule or route used. Biotherapy is now an established treatment modality in some cancers.

It is important to remember that rIL-2 is an immune drug, despite the fact that it was initially evaluated as a treatment for cancer. When these intellectual blinkers are abandoned, a host of additional potential applications become apparent. Some of these have been covered in this chapter.

Perhaps the most exciting prospect for the future is the gene therapy work of Rosenberg and colleagues. The human studies are at a very early stage, but they present new opportunities for both the patient and the physician. The goal, to provide optimal treatment with minimal morbidity, is one which has preoccupied cancer therapists for years. Many false starts have been made, but gene therapy, in some form, really looks a very promising concept.

As more basic work is carried out, our appreciation of the complex interactions which occur in the presence of IL-2 will undoubtedly contribute to a better use of these innovative molecules. In the absence of a complete understanding, there will always be a less than optimal results. Nevertheless, basic facts can be utilised now with some benefit.

This has already occured in patients with cancer, and is now being evaluated in other immune deficiency states, although some caution is required, particularly in HIV infections. The early data, however, are encouraging.

What is necessary is a pragmatic approach, and the appreciation that biotherapy is here to stay. Comparisons with early concepts of the magic bullet are completely inappropriate, and do a gross injustice to those who have worked so hard to unravel the puzzle. Recombinant technology has opened the biotherapy door. This is just the start of a great adventure in medicine, which will have a far-reaching impact on man.

References

1. Miller AB, Hoogstraten B, Staquet M, Winkler A. Reporting results of cancer treatment. Am J Cancer 1981; 47: 207–14.
2. Mulé JJ, Rosenberg SA. Interleukin-2: Pre-clinical trials. In: De Vita VT, Hellman S, Rosenberg SA, editors. Biologic Therapy of Cancer. London: JB Lippincott Co, 1991; 142–58.
3. Pinsky CM. Applicability of phase I trial results in the design of phase II and III biological response modifier trials. Cancer Treat Rep 1985; 69: 1171–3.
4. Jones M, Selby P, Bradley C, et al. Advanced renal cancer treated by interleukin-2 continuous infusion: comparison of survival to a matched control group. The 2nd Intl Symposium – Immunobiology of RCC, Cleveland Clinic 1991; 20: 136.
5. Lotze MT. Interleukin-2: Basic principles. In: De Vita VT, Hellman S, Rosenberg SA, editors. Biologic Therapy of Cancer. London: JB Lippincott Co, 1991; 123–41.
6. Winkelhake SL, Gauncy SS. Human recombinant interleukin-2 as an experimental therapeutic. Pharmacal Rev 1990; 42: 1–27.
7. Bradley EC, Carlin DA, Louie AC, et al. Antitumour response in patients with metastatic renal cell carcinoma is dependent upon regimen intensity. Proc ASCO 1989; 8: 519(abstract).
8. Collins FM, Morrison NE, Mantalbine V. Immune response to persistent mycobacterial infection in mice. Infect Immun 1978; 20: 430–8.
9. Lamoureux G, Poisson R. BCG and immunological anergy. Lancet 1974; 2: 989–91.
10. Colizzi V. In vivo and in vitro administration of interleukin-2 containing preparation reverses T-cell unresponsiveness in mycobacterium bovis BCG-infected mice. Infect Immun 1984; 45: 25–8.
11. Lundy J, Lovett EJ, Hamilton S, Conran P. Halothane, surgery, immunosuppression and artificial pulmonary metastases. Cancer 1978; 41: 827-30.
12. Lennard TWJ, Shenton BK, Borzotta A, et al. The influence of surgical operations on components of the immune system. Br J Surg 1985; 72.
13. Cochran AJ, Spilg WGS, Mackie RM, Thomas CE. Postoperative depression of tumour-directed cell-mediated immunity in patients with malignant disease. BMJ 1972; 4: 67–70.
14. Green DR, Faist E. Trauma and the immune response. Immunology Today 1988; 9: 253–5.
15. Lange PH, Hekmat K, Bosl G, et al. Accelerated growth of testicular cancer after cytoreductive surgery. Cancer 1980; 45: 1498–506.
16. Ausobsky JR, Evans M, Pollock AV. Levamisole and postoperative complications: a controlled clinical trial. Br J Surg 1980; 69: 447–8.
17. Yamaguchi K, Maeda S, Kitamura K. Prognostic factors in colorectal carcinoma: significance of peripheral T-lymphocytes. Int Surg 1989; 74: 232–9.
18. Carp N, Taylor D, Vollmer C, Weese J. Reversal of perioperative immunosuppression by recombinant interleukin-2 (rIL-2). Proc ASCO 1991; 10(abstract # 716).
19. Brevio F, Lissoni P, Tisi E, et al. Effects of a perioperative therapy with interleukin-2 on surgery-induced lymphocytopenia in cancer patients. Oncology 1992. In press.
20. Roth AD, Kirkwood JM. Neoclinical trials with interleukin-2: rationale for regional administration. Nat Immun Cell Growth Regul 1989; 8: 153–64.
21. Bubenik J. Local immunotherapy of cancer with interleukin-2. Immunol Lett 1989; 21: 267–74.
22. Eggermont AMN, Goey SH, Slingerland R, et al. Clinical and immunological evolution of intrapleural interleukin-2 in malignant pleural mesothelioma: a phase 1–2 study. Proc AACR 1991; 32(abstract # 1228).
23. Lemberskey B, Baldisseri M, Seski J, et al. Phase Ib study of intraperitoneal interleukin-2 for refractory ovarian cancer. Proc AACR 1990; 31(abstract # 1643).
24. Chapman PB, Hakes T, Gabrilove JL, et al. A phase I pilot study of intraperitoneal rIL-2 in ovarian cancer. Proc ASCO 1986; 5(abstract # 903).
25. Pizza GC, Severini G, Menniti D, et al. Tumour regression after intralesional injections of interleukin-2 in bladder cancer: preliminary report. Int J Cancer 1984; 34: 359–67.

26. Huland E, Huland H. Local continuous high dose interleukin-2: a new therapeutic model for the treatment of advanced bladder cancer. Cancer Res 1989; 49: 5469–74.
27. Velotti F, Tubaro A, Stoppacciaro A, et al. Local/regional recombinant interleukin-2 immunotherapy of tumours. Intra-arterial continuous infusion of rIL-2 in bladder cancer patients: a phase I study. Ann Ist Super Sanita 1990: 26: 3–4: 411–22.
28. Haaff EO, Catalona WJ, Ratliff TL. Detection of IL-2 in the urine of patients with superficial bladder tumours after treatment with intravesical BCG. J Urol 1986; 136: 970–4.
29. Tubaro A, Velotti F, Stoppacciaro A, et al. Intravesical immunotherapy of low stage bladder cancer with recombinant interleukin-2. Proc ASCO 1991; 10: 212(abstract # 710).
30. Bubenik J, Perlmann P, Indrova M, et al. Growth inhibition of an MC induced mouse sarcoma by TCGF (IL-2) containing preparations. Cancer Immunol Immunother 1983; 14: 205–6.
31. Bubenik J, Indrova M, Perlmann P, et al. Tumour inhibitory effects of TCGF/IL-2/containing preparations. Cancer Immunol Immunother 1985; 19: 57–61.
32. Bubenik J, Kieler J, Indrova M. Local treatment with human recombinant interleukin-2 inhibits growth of MC-induced sarcomas in syngeneic mice. Folia Biol 1986; 32: 209–11.
33. Forni G, Cavallo GP, Giovarelli M, et al. In: Homburger F, editor. Tumor immunotherapy by local injection of interleukin-2 and nonreactive lymphocytes: experimental and clinical results. Progress in Experimental Tumor Research. Basel: S. Karger, 1988: 187–212.
34. Cortesina G, De Stefan A, Giovarelli M, et al. Treatment of recurrent squamous cell carcinoma of the head and neck with low doses of interleukin-2 injected perilymphatically. J Cancer 1988; 62: 2482–5.
35. De Mulder PHM, Schornagel JH, Ruiter DJ, et al. A phase II study of perilymphatically injected recombinant interleukin-2 in locally far advanced, non-pretreated head and neck squamous cell carcinoma. NCI-EORTC Symposium on New Drugs in Cancer Therapy 1989.
36. Forni G, Giovarelli M, Jemma C, et al. Perilymphatic injections of cytokines: a new tool in active cancer immunotherapy – experimental rational and clinical findings. Ann Ist Sup Sanita 1989: 1–27.
37. Musiani P, De Campora E, Valitutti S, et al. Effect of low doses of interleukin-2 injected perilymphatically and peritumorally in patients with advanced primary head and neck squamous cell carcinoma. J Biol Response Mod 1989; 3: 571–8.
38. Rook AH, Masur H, Lane HC, et al. Interleukin-2 enhances the depressed natural killer and cytomegelovirus specific cytotoxic activities of lymphocytes from patients with the acquired immune deficiency syndrome. S Clin Invest 1983; 72: 398–403.
39. Ciobanu N, Welte K, Kruger G, et al. Defective T-cell response to PHA and mitogenic monoclonal antibodies in male homosexuals with acquired immune deficiency syndrome and its in vitro correction by interleukin-2. J Clin Immunol 1989; 3: 332–40.
40. Lotze MT, Robb RJ, Sharrow SO, et al. Systemic adminstration of interleukin-2 in humans. J Biol Response Mod 1984; 3: 375–482.
41. Clifford Lane H, Siegel JP, Rook AH, et al. Use of interleukin-2 in patients with acquired immune-deficiency syndrome. J Biol Response Mod 1984; 3: 512–6.
42. Mertelsmann R, Welte K, Sternberg C, et al. Treatment of immunodeficiency with interleukin-2: initial exploration. J Biol Response Mod 1984; 4: 483–90.
43. Volberding P, Moody DK, Beardslee D, et al. Therapy of acquired immune deficiency syndrome with recombinant interleukin-2. Aids Res Hum Retroviruses 1987; 3: 115–24.
44. Gotlieb MS, Wiefe PR, Mitsuyasu R. Immunotherapy of the acquired immune deficiency syndrome. In: Gallin JI, Fanci AS, editors. Advances in Host Defense Mechanism. New York: Raven Press, 1985; 5: 149–70.
45. Schwartz DH, Skowron G, Merigan TC. Safety and effects of interleukin-2 plus zidovudine in asymptomatic individuals infected with human immunodeficiency virus. J Acq Imm Def Synd 1991; 4: 11–23.
46. Kemeny M. Kaposi's sarcoma treated with long-term continuous IL-2 and AZT. Proc ASCO 1990; 9: 4(abstract # 10).
47. Mazza P, Bocchia M, Tumietto F, et al. rIL-2 in the treatment of lymphoma associated to HIV

infection. Preliminary report. VII International Conference on AIDS, Florence 1991; 274: 2369(abstract).
48. Nishioka M, Kagawa H, Shirai M, et al. Effects of human recombinant interleukin-2 in patients with chronic hepatitis B: a preliminary report. Am J Gastroenterol 1987; 82,5: 438–42.
49. Saibara T, Onishi S, Ito K. Clinical and immunological effects of recombinant interleukin-2 treatment in HBeAg-positive chronic hepatitis B. Viral Hepatitis and Liver Disease 1988: 879–83.
50. Ohta Y, Onji M, Kondoh H, et al. Recombinant interleukin-2 therapy for chronic hepatitis B virus infection. Viral Hepatitis and Liver Disease 1988: 884–6.
51. Kakumu S, Fuji A, Yoshioka K, et al. Pilot study of recombinant human interleukin-2 for chronic type b hepatitis. Hepatology 1988; 8: 3: 487–92.
52. Onji M, Kondoh H, Horiike N, et al. Effect of recombinant interleukin-2 on hepatitis B e antigen positive chronic hepatitis. Gut 1987; 28: 1648–52.
53. Bach N, Schaffner F, Lin SC. High-dose recombinant interleukin-2 for chronic viral hepatitis. Lancet 1989; II: 281.
54. Vogel W, Tilg H, Tratkiewicz J, et al. Natural interleukin-2 in chronic hepatitis B: phase I study. Hepatology 1989; 10: 4: 519(abstract).
55. Müller R, Schmidt HJ, Rahn A, et al. Recombinant interferon alfa-2b (IFN α-2b) and interleukin-2 (IL-2) in the treatment of chronic type B hepatitis. Symposium on Viral Hepatitis and its Treatment. The Present and the Future 1991.
56. Anderson G, Urban O, Fedorka-Cray P, et al. In: Chanock RM, Laner RA, Brown F, Ginsberg H, editors. Vaccines 87. Interleukin-2 and protective immunity in haemophilus pleuropneumonaie: preliminary studies. New York: Cold Spring Harbor Lab, Cold Spring Harbor, 1987: 22–6.
57. Nunberg JH, Doyle MV, York SM, York CJ. Interleukin-2 acts as an adjuvant to increase the potency of inactivated rabies virus vaccine. Proc Natl Acad Sci USA 1989; 86: 4240–3.
58. Kawamura H, Rosenberg SA, Berzofsky SA. Immunization with antigen and interleukin-2 in vivo overcomes Ir gene low responsiveness. J Exp Med 1985; 162: 381–6.
59. Meuer SC, Dumann H, Meyer zum Büschenfelde KH, Köhler H. Low-dose interleukin-2 induces systemic immune responses against HBsAg in immunodeficient non-responders to hepatitis B vaccination. Lancet 1989; I: 15–7.
60. Szmuness W, Stevens CE, Harley EJ, et al. Hepatitis B vaccine: demonstration of efficacy in a controlled clinical trial in a high-risk population in the United States. N Engl J Med 1980; 303: 833–41.
61. Meuer SC, Cooper DA, Hodgdon JC, et al. Identification of the antigen MHC receptor on human inducer T lymphocytes. Science 1983; 222: 1239–42.
62. Neidhart JA, Murphy SG, Hennick LA, Wise HA. Active specific immunotherapy of stage IV renal carcinoma with aggregated tumour antigen adjuvant. Cancer 1980; 46: 1128–34.
63. Hanna MG, Hoover HC. Active specific immunotherapy as an adjuvant to the treatment of metastatic solid tumours. In: Reif AE, Mitchell MS, editors. Immunity to Cancer. Orlando: Academic Press 1985: 429–40.
64. Hoover HC, Surdyke MG, Dangel RB, et al. Prospective randomised trial of adjuvant active specific immunotherapy for human colorectal cancer. Cancer 1985; 55: 1236–43.
65. Berd D, Maguire HC, Mastranigelo MJ. Induction of cell-mediated immunity to autologous melanoma cells and regression of metastases after treatment with a melanoma cell vaccine preceded by cyclosphosphamide. Cancer Res 1986; 46: 2572–7.
66. Bystryn JC, Jacobsen S, Harris M, et al. Preparation and characterisation of a polyvalent melanoma antigen vaccine. J Biol Response Mod 1986; 5: 211–24.
67. Houghton AN. Biological therapy of melanoma: Where do we go from here? Thirty-Fifth Annual Clinical Conference and Twenty-Fourth Annual Special Pathology Program – Advances in the Biology and Clinical Management of Melanoma, Houston, Texas 1991.
68. Mitchell MS, Kan-Mitchell J, Kempf RA, et al. Active specific immunotherapy for melanoma: phase I trial of allogeneic lysate and a novel adjuvant. Cancer Res 1988; 48: 5883–93.

69. Mitchell MS, Harel W, Kempf RA, et al. Active-specific immunotherapy for melanoma. J Clin Onc 1990; 8,5: 856–69.
70. Yron I, Wood TA, Spiess PJ, et al. In vitro growth of murine T cells v. the isolation and growth of lymphoid cells infiltrating syngeneic solid tumours. J Immunol 1980; 125: 238–45.
71. Lotze MT, Line BR, Mathisen DJ, et al. The in vivo distribution of autologous human and murine lymphoid cells grown in T cell growth factor (TCGF). Implications for the adoptive immunotherapy of tumours. J Immunol 1980; 125: 1487–93.
72. Rosenberg SA, Lotze MT, Muul LM, et al. Observations on the systemic administration of autologous lymphokine-activated killer cells and recombinant interleukin-2 to patients with metastatic cancer. N Engl J Med 1985; 25–19: 1485–92.
73. Rosenberg SA, Lotze MT, Yang JC, et al. Experience with the use of high dose bolus interleukin-2 in the treatment of 652 patients with cancer. Ann Surg 1989; 210: 474–85.
74. Rosenberg SA, Spiess P, Lafreniere R. A new approach to the adoptive immunotherapy of cancer with tumour infiltrating lymphocytes. Science 1986; 233: 1318–21.
75. Spiess PJ, Yang JC, Rosenberg SA. In vivo antitumour activity of tumour infiltrating lymphocytes expanded in recombinant interleukin-2. J Natl Cancer Inst 1987; 79: 1067–75.
76. Schwartzentruber DJ, Topalian SL, Mancini MJ, et al. Specific release of granulocyte-macrophage colony stimulating factor, tumour necrosis factor-a and IFN-α by human tumour infiltrating lymphocytes after autologous tumour stimulation. J Immunol 1991; 146: 153–64.
77. Fisher B, Packard BS, Read EJ, et al. Tumour localisation of adoptively transferred indium-111 labelled tumour infiltrating lymphocytes in patients with metastatic melanoma. J Clin Oncol 1989; 7: 250–61.
78. Griffith KD, Read EJ, Carrasquillo CS, et al. In vivo distribution of adoptively transferred indium-111 labelled tumour infiltrating lymphocytes and peripheral blood lymphocytes in patients with metastatic melanoma. J Natl Cancer Inst 1989; 81: 1709–17.
79. Rosenberg SA. The immunotherapy and gene therapy of cancer. J Clin Oncol 1992; 10,2: 180–99.
80. Miller AD, Buttimore C. Redesign of retrovirus packaging cell lines to avoid recombination leading to helper virus production. Mol Cell Biol 1986; 6: 2895–902.
81. Miller AD, Rosman GJ. Improved retroviral vectors for gene transfer and expression. Biotechniques 1989; 7: 980–6.
82. Rosenberg SA, Aebersold P, Corretta K, et al. Gene transfer into humans – Immunotherapy of patients with advanced melanoma using tumour-infiltrating lymphocytes modified by retroviral gene transduction. N Engl J Med 1990; 323: 570–8.
83. Carswell EA, Old LJ, Kassel RC, et al. An endotoxin-induced serum factor that causes necrosis of tumors. Proc Natl Acad Sci USA 1975; 72: 3666–70.
84. Wang AM, Creasy AA, Ladner MB, et al. Molecular cloning of the complementary DNA for human tumor necrosis factor. Science 1985; 228: 149–54.
85. Asher AL, Mulé JJ, Reichert CM, et al. Studies of the anti-tumor efficacy of systemically administered recombinant tumor necrosis factor against several murine tumors in vivo. J Immunol 1987; 138: 963–74.
86. McIntosh JE, Mulé JJ, Merino MJ, et al. Synergistic antitumor effects of immunotherapy with recombinant interleukin-2 and recombinant tumor necrosis factor-alpha. Cancer Res 1988; 48: 4011–7.
87. Blick MB, Sherwin SA, Rosenblum MG, Gutterman JU. A phase I trial of recombinant tumour necrosis factor in cancer patients. Proc ASCO 1986; 5(abstract # 14).
88. Chapman PB, Lester TJ, Casper, et al. Phase I study of recombinant tumour necrosis factor. Proc ASCO 1986; 5(abstract # 231).
89. Creagan ET, Kovach JS, Moertel CG, et al. A phase I clinical trial of recombinant human tumour necrosis factor. Cancer 1988; 62: 2467–71.
90. Tepper RI, Pattengale PK, Leder P. Murine interleukin-4 displays potent anti-tumor activity in vivo. Cell 1989; 57: 503–12.
91. Fearon ER, Pardoll DM, Itaya T, et al. Interleukin-2 production by tumor cells bypasses T

helper function in the generation of antitumor response. Cell 1990; 60: 397–403.
92. Gansbacher B, Zier K, Daniels B, et al. Interleukin-2 gene transfer into tumor cells abrogates tumorgenicity and induces protective immunity. J Exp Med 1990; 172: 1217–24.
93. Gansbacher B, Bannerji R, Daniels B, et al. Retroviral vector-mediated γ-interferon gene transfer into tumor cells generates potent and long lasting antitumor immunity. Cancer Res 1990; 50: 7820–5.
94. Jones M, Selby P, Bradley C, et al. Advanced renal cancer treated by interleukin-2 continuous infusion: comparison of survival to a matched control group. The 2nd Intl Symposium - Immunobiology of RCC, Cleveland Clinic 1991; 20: 136.
95. Parkinson DR. Interleukin-2: further progress through greater understanding. J Natl Ca Inst 1990; 82: 1374–6(editorial).
96. Atzpodien J, Korfer A, Evers P, et al. Low dose subcutaneous recombinant interleukin-2 in advanced human malignancy: a phase 2 outpatient study. Mol Biother 1990; 2: 18–26.
97. Atzpodien J, Korfer A, Franks CR, et al. Home therapy with recombinant interleukin-2 and interferon-a2b in advanced human malignancies. Lancet 1990; 335: 1509–12.
98. Sleijfer DTh, Janssen RAJ, Willemse PHB, et al. Low dose regimen of interleukin-2 for metastatic renal carcinoma. Lancet 1990; 335: 1522–3.
99. Herberman RB. LAK cells for the adoptive therapy of cancer. FORUM 1991; 1.2: 106–19.
100. Kilbourn RG, Gross SS, Jubran A, et al. NG-methyl-L-arginine inhibits tumor necrosis factor-induced hypotension: implications for the involvement of nitric oxide. Proc Natl Acad Sci USA 1990; 87: 3629–32.
101. Ohkubo C, Bigos D, Jain RK. Interleukin-2 induced leukocyte adhesion to the normal and tumor microvascular endothelium in vivo and its inhibition by dextran sulfate: implications for vascular leak syndrome. Cancer Res 1991; 51: 1561–3.
102. Lissoni P, Brivio F, Barni S, et al. Neuroimmunotherapy of human cancer with interleukin-2 and the neurohormone melatonin: its efficacy in preventing hypotension. Anticancer Res 1990; 10: 1759–62.

Index

FSC
www.fsc.org
MIX
Papier aus verantwortungsvollen Quellen
Paper from responsible sources
FSC® C105338

If you have any concerns about our products,
you can contact us on
ProductSafety@springernature.com

In case Publisher is established outside the EU,
the EU authorized representative is:
Springer Nature Customer Service Center GmbH
Europaplatz 3, 69115 Heidelberg, Germany

Printed by Libri Plureos GmbH
in Hamburg, Germany